The Pilates Healing Bible

The Pilates
Healing Bible

Tone your body through exercise
that strengthens and conditions
the muscles and improves focus,
comfort, and clarity

Melissa Cosby

**CHARTWELL
BOOKS, INC.**

A QUANTUM BOOK

This edition published in 2013 by
CHARTWELL BOOKS, INC.
A division of BOOK SALES INC.,
276 Fifth Avenue, Suite 206
New York, New York 10001
USA

ISBN 13: 978-0-7858-3066-5

Produced by
Quantum Publishing Ltd
The Old Brewery
6 Blundell Street
London N7 9BH

QUMPLHB

Assistant Editor: Jo Morley
Editors: Hazel Eriksson and Sam Kennedy
Production Manager: Rohana Yusof
Publisher: Sarah Bloxham

Designed by Stonecastle Graphics
Studio photography by Marcos Bevilacqua
Models: Stephanie Owen and Xavier Serra

Printed in China by Midas Printing
International Ltd.

Quantum would like to thank and acknowledge
the following for supplying the pictures
reproduced in this book:

© Shutterstock: Lisa A 14; Action Sports
Photography 31; Andresr 22, 37; Zai Aragon
27; area381 33; auremar 15; ESTUDI M6 34;
Sunny Forest 11; Antonio Guillem 26; holbox
20, 21; Kzenon 216; Aleksandr Markin 7, 25;
michaeljung 35; Christopher Edwin Nuzzaco 8;
Andrey_Popov 24, 32; simonalvinge 17; Anatoli
Styf 29; Yellowj 30; Arman Zhenikeyev 13;
6348103963 18.

© Getty Images: Michael Rougler 19.

All other photographs and illustrations are the
copyright of Quantum Publishing Ltd

While every effort has been made to credit
contributors, Quantum would like to apologize
should there have been any omissions or errors.

Contents

Introduction

Welcome to *The Pilates Healing Bible*. This book aims to give you some great workout tools, as well as some "how-to" skills to help you employ them well. Using them will take up no more than a few minutes of your time, and reward you with more focus, comfort, and clarity—from the moment you wake, throughout your working day, and into the evening, as they ease you toward a good night's sleep.

Opposite: Pilates is a valuable part of any fitness routine to create balance and strength and leave you feeling refreshed and at ease.

The drills in this book are warm-ups, stretches, and relaxation routines to help you prepare for a full Pilates practice. Some are formulated to be done at your desk, others on the floor at home, and there is also a classical Pilates mat routine.

Pilates is a blend of disciplines. It is informed by gymnastics, Olympic weightlifting, tai chi and everything else that piqued the curiosity of its inventor, Joseph Pilates. It is a method that seeks to rebalance the body, enabling it to achieve complex whole movements, and can be applied to any activity you want to work on. The field of physical therapy is providing more and more evidence that whole body movements are the key to boosting overall competency in both daily activity and sports. If a therapist diagnoses a weak muscle that inhibits your movements and then suggests an exercise that focuses simply on strenthening *that* muscle, you still may not improve, even though the culprit muscle has been strengthened. *Until you keep practicing with more attention to all aspects of that movement, you are not focusing on the whole picture.*

So, use the control and self-mastery you will learn here to enhance or inspire all your sporting goals, be they running, football, CrossFit, swimming, dancing, or any other endeavor!

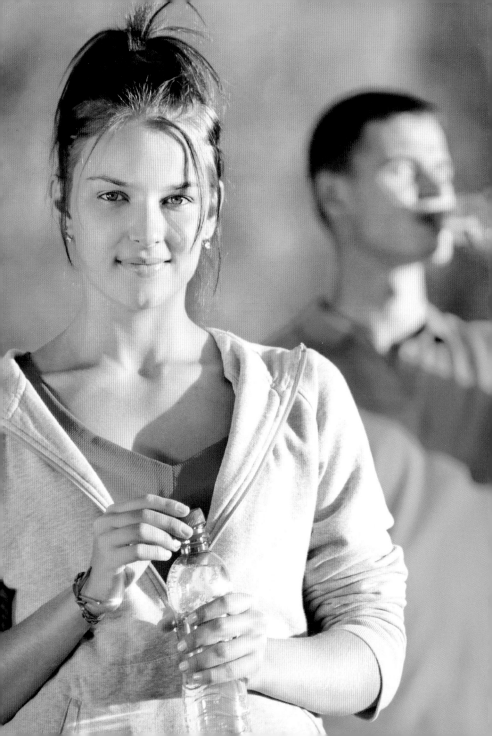

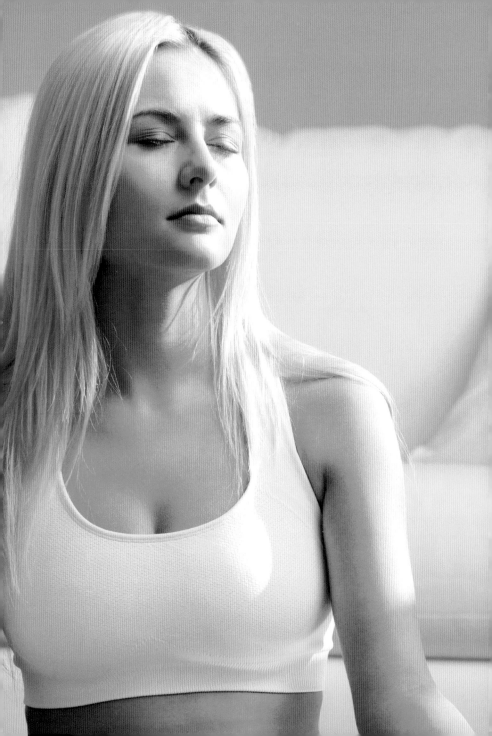

Pilates and Healing

There are various definitions of "healing" including "to restore to health or soundness", "to set right," and "to make whole." In a physical scenario, we can say that the process of restoring to health an unbalanced, damaged, or painful part of the body and reintegrating it into a fully functioning, pain-free body would be considered healing. In effect, this is what Joseph Pilates advocated many years ago—that by paying attention to all aspects of your health and how they fit together, a strong, dynamic, and flexible body and mind will result.

Mindfulness

"That single aspect which, when practiced, can bring together mind and body." "Mindfulness," as is it commonly referred to today, is based on Buddhist meditation, but the process is not inherently religious at all.

In a nutshell, mindfulness is paying attention to what is happening right now, both within and around you. Importantly, mindfulness should come before any judgment, interpretation of, or action upon a situation.

You could say that being mindful is the counter to being on autopilot or operating from habit. So many of our actions in normal day-to-day life are habitual. We don't notice how, when, why—or, even *that* we do them. Think about your daily commute to work. Can you have a conversation while listening to the radio and driving at the same time? If you're an experienced driver, the answer is probably "yes." You have a goal in mind (drive to work), and your unconscious sets about the task, leaving your conscious mind to free-wheel onto anything else of its choosing.

Our habits of posture, breath, and movement tend to receive the same levels of attention. We sit at our desks, get in and out of the car, carry the kids, and even lift weights the same way we did yesterday and the day before. And that's fine, so long as the habits we have are serving us and our baseline posture. But developing mindfulness allows us to attune ourselves more closely to our bodies, gives us the opportunity to fix things that may be getting out of kilter, and can go on to help us achieve much more.

Our bodies are both the genesis of, and the storehouse for, the results of our thoughts, feelings, and actions; that's why our posture says so much about us! Focusing on the body can be a great way to learn something from scratch, as well as a means of teaching ourselves how to get better at what we think we can do already. When we hit a plateau in our skills or strength, paying more attention to the *how* of a thing can accelerate our mastery of it.

Mindfulness can also help when we encounter things we think we *can't* do. It challenges our preconceptions and fears, helps us focus on what is actually happening, and enables us to try something new and see what happens. So, if you get stuck when exercising, be aware of your sensations, remember the goal of the exercise, hone your focus, and see if you're able to continue. Usually you can, and often you will surprise yourself.

Below: Imagining yourself to be somewhere beautiful and calm can be a great aid to finding a moment for yourself.

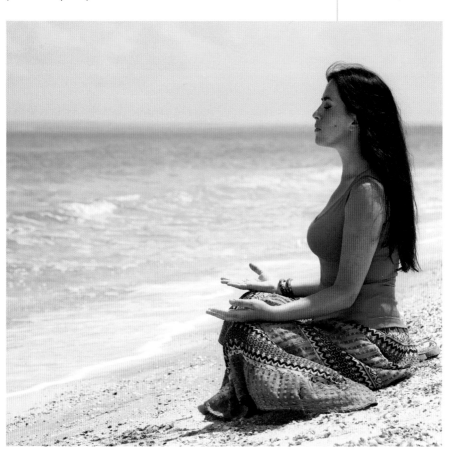

Mindfulness in Action

So how do we *do* mindfulness? The word is often translated as "awareness"—a close match but not the entire picture. Take the previous example of driving to work. Being aware of the fact *that* you are driving is only part of the picture. A "mindful" account would also take in *how* and *why* you're driving as you are, and the realization that you can change your way of doing so if you choose.

The same principle exists in relation to posture, breathing, and exercise. Thinking that you should improve these is a good initial step...but not very useful if it ends there. Instead, get purposeful about what your body is doing and how you'd like to alter it, use it to explore how you might reach your goal, focus on that end, and you'll have everything rolling efficiently (if sometimes slowly) in the right direction. It doesn't require force and fight, just clear intention, well applied.

When teaching class, I invite clients to "arrive" before we start exercising. Often this only takes a few breaths, but sometimes I notice breathing patterns that are so arrested, congested, and constrained that loading them any further will just increase the underlying tension. In such situations, I allow a little more "settling-in" time.

The same thing can happen when you're working out on your own, and a voice in your head says: "I just need to get through this, as I've only got x minutes..." However, you will reap far more benefit by doing fewer exercises in a better frame of mind and body—of which your breath will be a great indicator.

How many times have you gone to a class and been told to "drop your shoulders" when you don't understand what that means, let alone how to do it? This is an example of not being "in your body." Knowing where you are in space, and where you are holding tension in various parts of your body, is essential to the practice of mastering your body and your mind too.

Try it now by seeing if you can describe the sensations in and around your shoulders as you read. What qualities do they have? Are they hard or soft? As you move them, do they conjure up a feeling, a sound, or an image? Remember that there's no correct way of conveying your sensations. Everyone has very different ways of feeling their body and the more latitude you give yourself when learning to listen to your body, the easier you'll find it.

Below: Mindfulness will help you to relax and live in the moment.

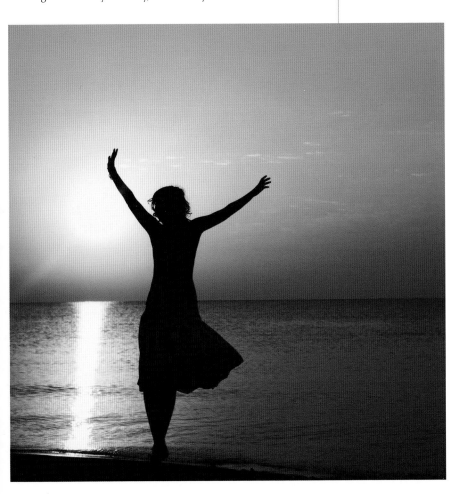

Your Still Point—An Exercise in Mindfulness

Become aware of your mind and its activity—its thoughts. Know that it is your mind's job to create thoughts and that they are separate from you. By understanding that your thoughts are separate makes it easier to be unconcerned by their content.

As your thoughts come and go, you may notice more distance between what you perceive as "you" and the thoughts themselves. Breathe.

Notice your body as you watch your thoughts from a distance. Does it feel quiet? Buzzing? Open? Tight? Relaxed? Peaceful? Is one part of your body clearer than another? Observe a single sensation or area of your body, and let the intensity of the other parts fade into the background. Find a couple of words that best describe this feeling or body part, or take a "feeling photo" of that set of sensations.

Below: Good form in exercise requires awareness of both your internal and external environment.

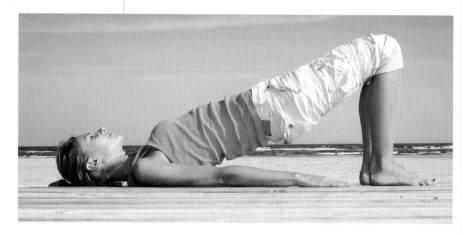

Now bring your awareness to your breath. First, just observe it as it is. After a minute, gently coax your breath into a smoother rhythm. Perhaps count to four as you breathe in, and four again as you breathe out. Do this for another minute.

Now check the sensations you were observing before. Describe them to yourself: Not what you think about them or what you think they mean—just the sensations themselves. "My breath is super slow." "My arms are heavy." "My legs tingle."

Gently open your eyes. Do you lose your internal awareness as your senses are flooded with external input?

When we start mindful exercise, we often have to close our eyes and shut off the stimuli of the external world so we can stay attuned to the internal ones. That's fine. Ultimately you'll be able to have a simultaneous handle on how you are in yourself and how you are in the world.

Until that time, play between the two. When you get too involved in external activity, close your eyes, notice your breath, and follow it all the way in and all the way out. If you're exercising, feel the sensations of the exercise in action.

Below: Closing your eyes can help you to turn your focus inward.

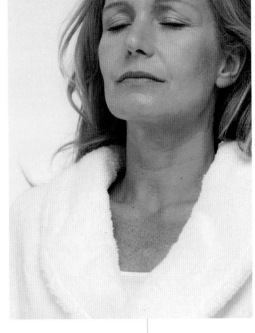

What you're doing is a way of self-regulating, and you can use it in many ways. It may serve simply to calm down the voices in your head all vying for attention, so you can focus clearly on the next thing that needs doing.

In the context of this book, this is healing—bringing your physical and mental self to a communal focus.

15

Mindfulness in Pilates

A key element of Pilates is the recognition that what we do with the body has an effect on the mind, and vice versa. Like yoga, it focuses on "mindful" activity and movement.

Where to gaze, how to breathe, ideal body alignment, duration of pose or number of repetitions, and even how to eat, clean, sleep, stand and walk—all these are prescribed by the Pilates system. And just as with yoga, it isn't necessary for you to subscribe to every aspect of the discipline: I encourage you to find your own ideal, and choose the parts that are beneficial to you.

Pilates is based on paying attention to everything relating to your life and health via its exercises, the way you do them, what you eat, and how you sleep. At times, these essentials have been overlooked, but you have only to consider the characteristics of mindfulness set out by the system to understand their comprehensiveness. In order to move your limbs, breathe, and co-ordinate you have to know where you are in space, and make a decision about where you want to go. You get there by being in the present moment and staying engaged in the process. You don't need to *think* about being mindful; you attain mindfulness by executing the Pilates principles.

Why do we go slower at the beginning? We need to be aware of what is actually happening to us as we carry out the exercises. Then we have choices. Do I need to make the movements smaller? Can I reach more, breathe deeper? As we get more proficient in smaller, slower movements, we can increase the speed, size, and repetitions. By paying attention, and resisting the mental temptation to "Go!" at the cost of control, we'll be able to progress further and faster.

You should start out slow and small to avoid overtaxing your system while you're learning. As you progress, begin to try harder versions of each exercise—adding pace, range, or weight will give you a new set of things to consider!

I love forward motion, progress ,and improvement, and I know that the best way to achieve them is by staying in balance and challenging my comfort level. So when you're applying these principles, stay a moment where it's uncomfortable or difficult and get some information about how that feels. Then decide if it's useful to carry on—and how best to modify what you have been doing.

Below: The mental freedom and relaxation from a good workout is linked to the increase in your physical strength and skill.

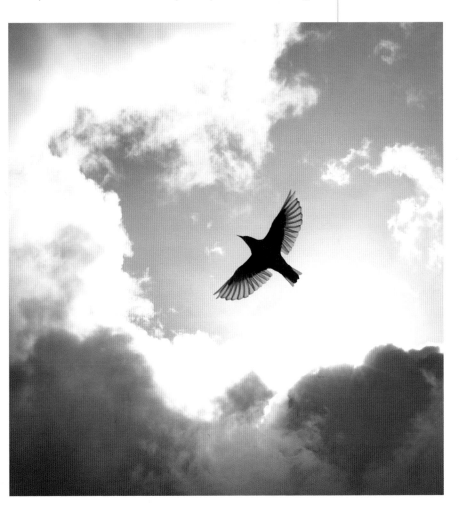

What is Pilates?

Pilates as we now know it was the brainchild and life's work of Joseph Pilates (1883-1967). Born near Düsseldorf, Germany, he was a sickly child, suffering from rickets, asthma, and rheumatic fever.

Since his mother was a naturopath and father an award-winning gymnast, it's probable that Joseph would have been taken to local spas, and encouraged to follow the exercise regimes that were then commonly prescribed to people in poor health.

As a child, he latched onto physical training to increase his strength and fitness. By the age of 14 his body was so well developed that he was posing for anatomy charts. As a teenager he skied, dived, and practiced gymnastics. He continued to study eastern physical arts and the mind-body connection through karate, yoga, and Zen meditation.

In 1912, Joseph Pilates moved to England, where he was a professional boxer and self-defense instructor. Two years later, at the

Right: Modern Pilates is recognized as an ideal form of exercise for ballet dancers.

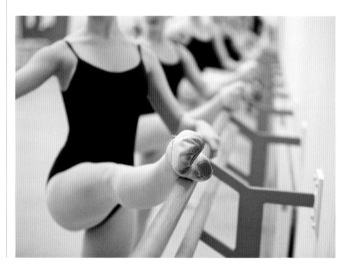

beginning of World War One, he was interned as an enemy alien, and it was during this period that he began teaching his own methods for attaining physical fitness.

Toward the end of the war, he was moved to the Isle of Man, where he assisted with the rehabilitation of injured hospital patients by devising exercises they could perform in their beds, using resistance apparatus created by removing the bedsprings and attaching them to the bed-heads. Modern Pilates equipment adopts the same principles.

Joseph relocated to New York after the war. He and his wife Clara (whom he'd met on the voyage from England) opened a studio on 8th Avenue opposite the New York City Ballet, and became closely involved with training some of the city's leading ballet dancers and choreographers. Through his work with them, his own work became less focused on developing boxing-style strength, incorporated more flow and smoother transitions, and eventually gained a reputation as an exercise form for rehabilitating dancers and athletes.

In 1934 Pilates published a booklet about his method, *Your Health*. It set out to change the lives of ordinary people, warning them of the dangers of a sedentary lifestyle. Eleven years later, he co-authored *Return to Life Through Contrology* with

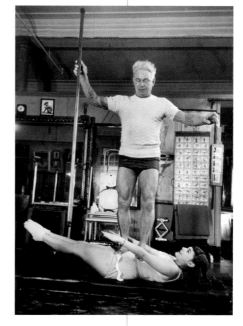

W.J. Miller. This book expanded his philosophies and principles of exercise, and included detailed descriptions of exercises to be practiced daily at home.

Pilates' approach was in line with yoga and eastern traditions, and promoted the idea that mental and physical health are interrelated. His system was an all-inclusive one, intended to teach people that their bodies' wellbeing was affected by how they thought, what they ate, how they breathed, and how they moved.

Above: Joseph Pilates embodied the principle that mental and physical wellbeing are interrelated.

19

Pilates Today

Pilates is perceived in many different ways today: as the exercise of choice for those who don't want to do any exercise, as rehabilitation, as a sexy choice for movie stars, or as a strong workout that will last its disciples a lifetime and provide them with ever-changing day-to-day challenges.

In classical or "authentic" Pilates studios, the only routines practiced are the ones its creator himself is believed to have followed. They can be excellent when taught by an experienced and nuanced instructor. However, problems can arise when teachers try to cram a student's body into the system without adequate preparation or understanding, and I have been hurt in such classes.

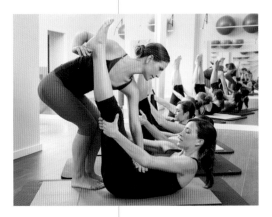

Other studios have taken the system, broken it down into its principles, and devised a physiotherapeutic model based on Pilates. This can be great if you need to iron out a kink or heal an injury, but can be stifling for growth if you're with a trainer who engenders fear of unsupervised movement. I've been there too, and have ended up getting so tense trying to make my movements perfect that I achieved nothing.

A third type of studio blends Pilates exercises with cardio or circuit training to create a hybrid. These classes can make for a great workout in terms of sweat and energy, but I have seen participants moving without attention to form, control, precision, or focus on breath.

Above: In a class you will benefit from the personal advice of a qualified instructor.

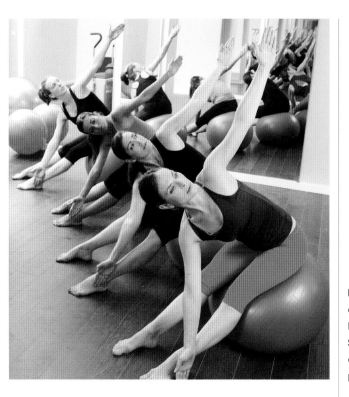

Left: There are many different types of Pilates class available. Some are mat-based and others use various pieces of equipment.

All these approaches have something valuable to offer if you know what you're looking for, and if you have enough of what they don't provide represented elsewhere in your exercise life. Some so-called Pilates classes involve adaptations that are such significant departures from what Pilates is all about, that it would be better if they were given a different name. Beginners, who are, by definition, uninitiated, will be misled, and may end up hurting themselves, if they don't get the proper type of Pilates training.

So if you're looking for either a mat class or an equipment-based studio experience, look around, ask around, speak to a number of teachers. Ask them questions about why they take the approach they do. Make sure that you get what version of Pilates you're looking for to meet your needs or achieve your goals.

21

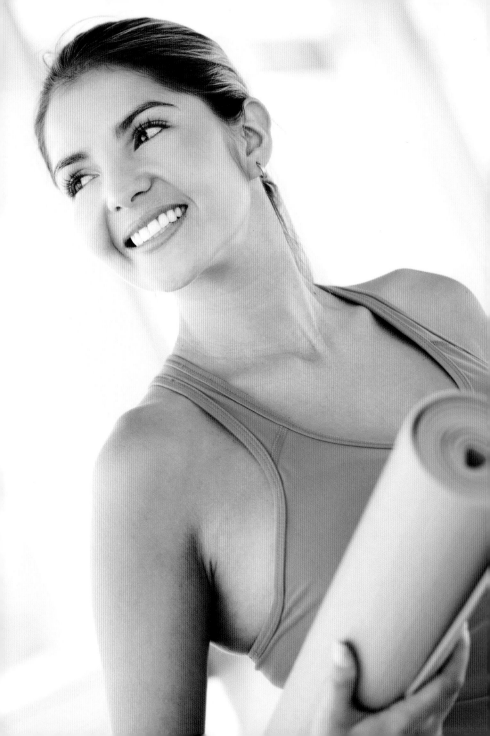

Getting Started

The goal of this book is to teach the cornerstone of mindful Pilates practice; a purposeful and peaceful mental state. This will allow you to make the most of the exercise routines.

The routines in this book do not require equipment; some can even be done at your desk! By using these routines, you will find that there is room for Pilates in your daily life.

Principles of Pilates

Joseph Pilates, while having clear guiding principles to his work, did not come up with the definition of "Pilates" we know and roughly agree on today. It was in 1980 that Philip Friedman and Gail Eisen published the first modern book on the subject. Entitled *The Pilates Method of Physical and Mental Conditioning*, it contained six "Principles of Pilates": **Concentration**, **Control**, **Center**, **Flow**, **Precision**, and **Breathing**.

Below: Get the most out of your routine by practicing the basic principles of Pilates.

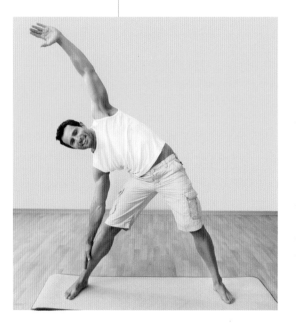

These principles have been adopted and adapted by the Pilates community. I've added two additional ones. **Ease**: because it's possible to become so preoccupied with getting everything perfect that you'll forget to breathe. **Agency**: Because taking ownership of your physical life is empowering. I believe that when you make any practice your own, it'll stay with you much longer than something imposed from the outside. If we're going to use this system to help us self-regulate, then we must be able to adapt it to our needs.

It's only possible to grasp these principles in waves at first. You can concentrate all the time, but only on one or two things until your nervous system starts to wire in the movement patterns. Prior to that, you'll get a bit of center, a bit of precision—

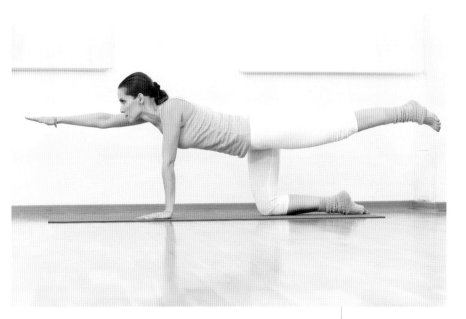

then things get rigid—so you remember to flow—and you wobble a bit. That's ok, it's an important part of learning. So relax. Have a laugh if you just fell over; make the movement a bit smaller or slower, and try again.

By instructing students to concentrate, and then giving them specific breath and body cues about what to concentrate on, teamed with markers ("This goes *there*, like *that*..."), Joseph Pilates was teaching mindfulness.

Breath is the bridge between consciousness and unconscious as it can be controlled by both systems. Control is both something you possess, and something that's evident from the outside—so it's a perfect marker. Flow is a refined example of control; precision too.

We can say that the learning process is roughly as follows: Working from your center and being precise with your movements, you will have control over your body and it will flow. Co-ordinate this with breath and you will have control over your mind too. Further ideas also born of mindfulness—**Effort, Listening, Intention,** and **Self-reliance**—can also be applied to each of these principles.

Above: The principles of Pilates teach us control by working from our center and being precise in our movements.

25

Breathing

"Above all, learn how to breathe correctly."

Breathing is important in the Pilates method. Joseph Pilates likened it to "bodily house-cleaning with blood circulation," and placed great importance on increasing oxygen intake and circulating oxygenated blood to every part of the body. He considered forced exhalation as the key to full inhalation, and advised people to squeeze out their lungs as if they were wringing out a wet towel.

D espite the fact that breathing is a fundamental Pilates principle, focusing doggedly on it can hinder the flow of movement. One simple cue to keep you moving is to exhale where there is effort and then direct the inhale into the back and sides of the lower ribcage. As your familiarity with each exercise increases, you will be able to deepen your practice with increased focus on your breath, and awareness of the nuances that breathing can have on mood and movement.

Right: Take your time when breathing and feel the conscious connection between your breath and relaxation.

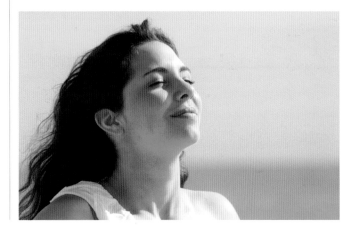

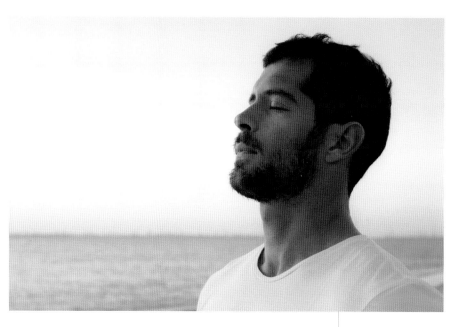

If the effort phase is not clear in any given exercise, or there is effort in both directions, employ the principle of inhaling when the spine is extending (bending backwards), and exhaling when the spine is flexing (bending forward).

Initially, focus on keeping the breath flowing, and keeping your neck and shoulders relaxed throughout the moment. Many of us struggle with this and lift our shoulders up to assist filling the lungs. To learn how to breathe more fully, and with less effort, here's a mental visualization technique which may help you:

Think of your lungs as two deflated wrinkly balloons side by side in your ribcage. As you slowly inhale they start to fill. They will expand simultaneously in all directions, front, sides, back, top, and bottom. When you exhale, think of the balloons deflating. It's easy. The air just falls out, with your lungs deflate again as the air goes.

Even when we are exercising and need to be stable, we still need to be able to breathe. Be careful of locking your ribcage down with your abdominal muscles. If, when you are moving you can't get a breath in, reconsider the amount of effort you are using.

Above: Relax your neck and send your breath down and to the sides of your ribs.

27

Centering

When most of us consider movement, we think about what our arms and legs are doing, but even when the exercise or movement might involve arms and legs, they will have little power if not connected into the torso.

Opposite: The center is the focal point of the Pilates method.

The idea that power and stability translate to rigidity is a misconception. Your center is not a rigid place, but one moving in accordance with gravity, planes of movement, and limb placement. Rather, it must be ever flexible, and also ever responsive to the demands of your life, be those sport or exercise, or just the hustle and bustle of daily life.

In a Pilates class you will often hear the term "Powerhouse". It is a commonly used term to describe the center of strength and stability in the trunk. Efficient use of the powerhouse offers a solid foundation for all movement. The primary powerhouse includes the muscles and fascia in and extending from the abdominals, lower back, pelvis, and hips. These muscles work together to form a supportive corset for your trunk. The Powerhouse stabilizes us, creates the big moves we make, and gives those moves their dynamic strength.

Even though the powerhouse is considered to be in the lower part of the torso, how we connect our arms to it via back, chest, and abdominals is as important as how our legs hook in through the pelvis for channeling power and grace into our movements.

Pilates beginners need to think in terms of using this powerhouse right away. It gives us the energy, stability, strength, and control to move into the intermediate and advanced Pilates exercises.

Being physically centered can give rise to a feeling of security, and an ability to remain unruffled by that which is going on around us; it can act as an anchor in our lives. With this foundation we are prepared mentally and physically for what life throws at us. We are stronger, more grounded, calmer.

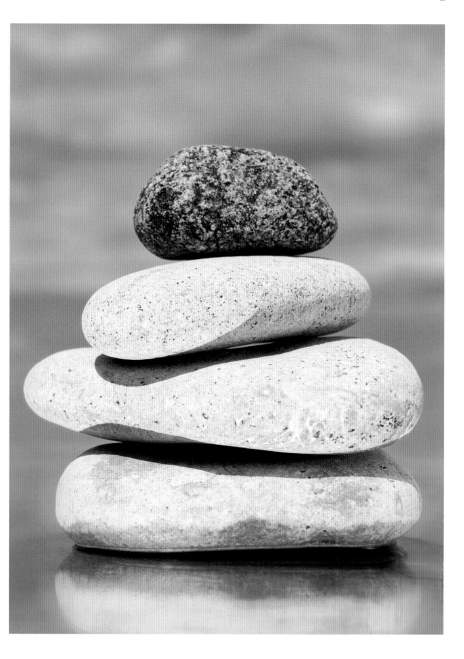

Concentration

"You have to concentrate on what you're doing all the time. And you must concentrate on your entire body for smooth movements."

Pilates demands intense focus. If you aren't paying attention to what you are doing, the results you seek will remain hidden. Concentration may be needed, to some degree, for almost any task in daily life, but Pilates absolutely depends upon it and, to Pilates practitioners, "concentration" represents not simply a careful consideration of what *should* be happening, but also the application of focused intention in order to *make* it happen.

The pursuit of Pilates, and the constant striving and refining it involves, can be a lifetime's work. A study in 2006 indicated that the *way* its exercises are done is more important than the exercises themselves—and at the Oregon Health & Science University's Parkinson Center, its benefits have been studied as a way of alleviating the poor movement control, tremors, and other symptoms of Parkinson's Disease.

Below: Concentrating on your mind and body will enable you to perform smoother movements with greater effect.

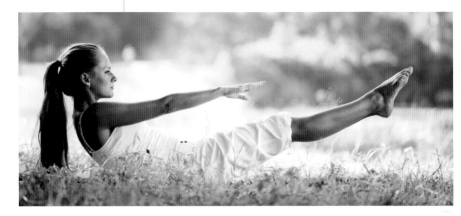

Control

"Nothing about the Pilates Method is haphazard. The reason you need to concentrate so thoroughly is so you can be in control of every aspect of every moment."

This is mindfulness in movement. If you know where your body is in space, what it is doing, and what you want it to be doing, you have more chance of teaching it to go there. And you have to stay mentally and physically engaged as you perform the movement to remain in control of it. This doesn't happen overnight. It takes repetition of movements to make them second nature; and they must usually start small and slow before they can gradually become faster, larger, and more powerful.

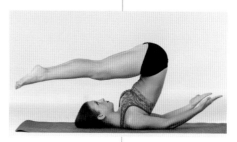

A controlled movement is obvious and beautiful when you see it—and Pilates requires that its practitioners should be in control of their movements at every moment while exercising. Its insistence on this has led to its widespread use as a rehabilitation tool for injured sportsmen and women, so many of whose injuries are caused by wild or rapid (uncontrolled) movements.

Above: All aspects of your body are involved in controlling complex movements.

All Pilates exercises are aimed at being full body exercises. There may be some primary moving parts, but the rest of the body is stabilizing, anchoring or opposing the movement. When it can work skillfully with and against resistance, the body has options; and when its small and large muscle groups are able to co-operate eccentrically and concentrically, balance and co-ordination are enhanced.

As Joseph Pilates put it himself, "The Pilates Method teaches you to be in control of your body and not at its mercy"—and its principles apply to every aspect of movement, not just inside the studio but also throughout everyday life.

Ease

"Physical fitness can neither be achieved by wishful thinking nor outright purchase."

We all work too hard, and often aren't aware of our energy levels, or how to conserve or replenish them. Once we've decided to exercise, we tend to choose one of three approaches: Getting the exercises done as hard and fast as possible, completing them in the minimum amount of time; daydreaming our way through the motions, in the vain hope that by approximating the prescribed body placements (and thereby "doing our exercises") we'll feel better; or working so hard that we almost combust. After all, by putting in three times the effort, the results must surely be three times better! (Not true, of course...)

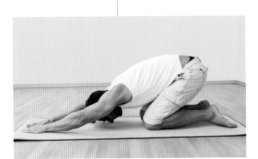

Above: Using just enough energy for the exercise at hand and no more will give you better overall results.

Going for any of the options above can be an indication that you're overloaded. You need to find a middle ground where just enough effort, applied in just the right way, will give the best results. This may mean careful selection of your exercises, or a change in your approach to them. It usually doesn't mean doing no exercises at all. Even when you're exhausted, a little gentle movement and connected breathing can set you up for a far better, deeper sleep than you'd achieve by falling straight into bed. The good news is that all this is something that you can learn with regular practice. Keep asking yourself questions about your approach. Can you do a particular exercise with the same intention but less effort? Sometimes, reducing the amount of what I call "noise" in my approach allows me to work harder, and at the end of a session, I will enjoy a quieter sense of achievement and fulfillment.

Flow

"Contrology is designed to give you suppleness, natural grace, and skill that will be unmistakably reflected in the way you walk, play, and work."

History has it that Joseph Pilates' method changed as a result of working with dancers, coming to prioritize smooth movements and grace in each exercise. But it's not just dancers for whom this flow is important. The principle of flow and rythmn speak to ideal human movement. We find it more soothing to move with flow; it is also more efficient and ironically more powerful, though it looks like less effort.

Flowing movement is wonderful for the soft tissues of the body. Glide in connective tissue represents health, encouraging flexibility, ease in joints and even distribution of forces throughout the body. Rhythm serves as a pump too, regulating the nervous system as well as the musculo-skeletal one.

Flow for Pilates, was about efficiency. His method aims for elegant sufficiency of movement, creating flow through the use of appropriate transitions between exercises, and general attention to detail when moving. Indeed Pilates' principle carried out into life outside the studio where he believed in the usefulness of creating the most efficient and simple ways of doing all daily tasks.

Below: Pilates exercises are intended to flow into each other to create flexibility and build strength.

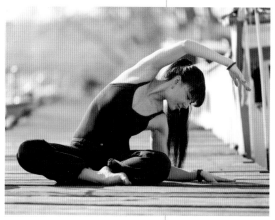

33

Precision

"Concentrate on the correct movements each time you exercise, lest you do them improperly and thus lose all the vital benefits of their value."

P recision is essential to Pilates. The aim is to perform one precise and ideal movement, rather than many unfocused ones. As Pilates himself put it: "A few well-designed movements, properly performed in a balanced sequence, are worth hours of doing sloppy calisthenics or forced contortion." Eventually, this precision should become second nature, and carry over into everyday life as grace and economy of movement.

Below: Precision is essential if you are to gain the most benefit from the movements.

Obviously you need control to be precise. Precision clarifies "where" you're doing "what." You should be asking yourself: "Where does this exercise start and finish? How big can I make it?" And if you experience discomfort or other problems, there may be ways to counter them: "My back hurts and I have to bend my knees a little, but then I go a bit soft. Ah—but if I lift my legs by just one centimeter, I can do the exercise strongly with no pain." It's essential to practice this kind of precision: The precision of knowing what the exercise is trying to give you, what you can do and exactly how you can do it.

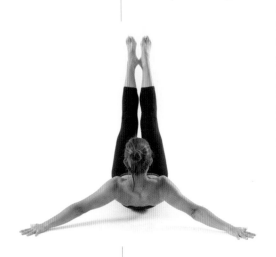

If you suffer from pain due to poor postural habits, you must start to learn exactly when those sensations go away. Ask yourself, for example, "If my neck feels stressed when I'm at the computer keyboard, how do I move my elbows to make it comfortable?" This kind of precision is essential because, if you don't figure out why undesirable sensations are happening, you'll be uncertain about how they can be changed. And remember, you're doing Pilates not just for the time you're on the mat; you want its effects to filter through to your everyday life.

Your journey here is one of learning. That includes figuring out what feels good and bad, within safe parameters. There's so much to remember in any given moment when you're learning something new, so don't set the bar too high by making an exercise too difficult and striving too hard for perfection, or you'll fall into the trap of "constipating" your movement (a nasty, but appropriate expression)— or, even worse, giving up because "I can't do it right, so what's the point?"

Other the other hand: half the time, when we think we can't do something, we can. So I ask youto challenge yourself and be inspired. Try taking one exercise a day a bit further than you intended. If you can't, scale back, as before, but I know you'll be stronger for the next attempt.

Below: Perform the movements precisely and in a balanced, rhythmic sequence.

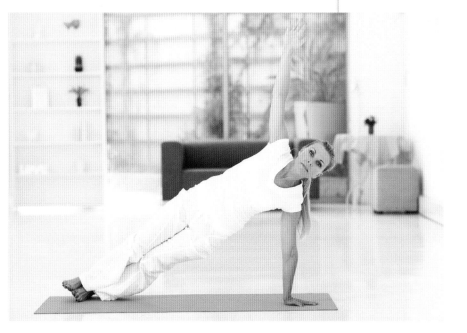

Your Pilates Practice

All you require to get started with the exercises in this book is a moment to get your head in the right space, and a few more moments to carry out the movements themselves.

Opposite: No matter who you are or what level of fitness or experience of Pilates you have, just make a start and adapt the exercises to your pace and requirements. You will soon be feeling the benefits of adding this routine to your life.

You'll need either your chair and desk at work, or a soft mat to protect your spine at home. If you have a carpeted floor, or a hardy spine and knees, you won't even need a mat! We want there to be no reason for you to "not move." Ever. Therefore, this book is designed to provide some loosening and limbering tools for you to use wherever you are, enabling you to de-stress your body and start obtaining the benefits of Pilates.

Remember the principle of beginning small and slow, and building either the speed or the size of the exercise as you feel comfortable. These exercises should not "hurt", but leave you with an agreeable, "worked-out" feeling. If they do hurt, stop. Re-assess your form, size and speed, and see if the feeling changes. This is where all the "awareness" we've been discussing becomes invaluable: It will help you to differentiate "good" sensations from "Uh-uh, something doesn't feel right" ones. And don't be alarmed by either! If changing your form, size, and speed doesn't make things feel better, that particular exercise is not for you today...and if it doesn't feel good again next time, go see a professional for a helping hand.

Choose a time of day for a longer routine and try to make it just that—a routine. You'll feel its benefit, and won't get so easily pushed off-track. For the shorter routines, grab a minute, whenever you have one, just to move. "Small and often" periods of exercise will help to keep you oiled up and ready for whatever life can throw at you.

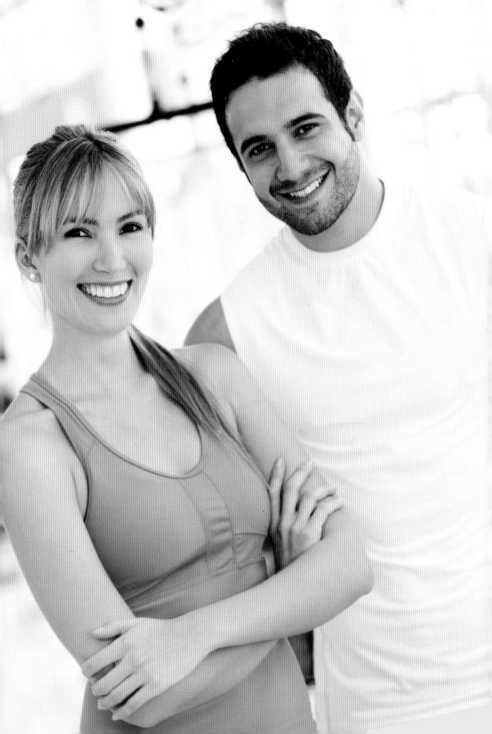

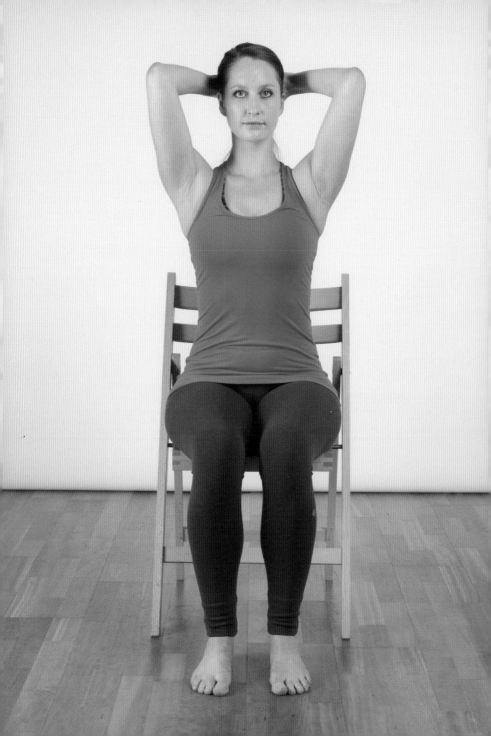

At Your Desk Routine: Stressed-Out Shoulders

Many people appreciate Pilates because of its close relationship to good posture. Even when you are stuck at your desk, there are principles you can use to make sure the hours spent there do not translate into a lifetime habit of slump, tension, and pain. Do the routine a couple of times and you will soon find the movements that immediately make a difference to you. Make sure you incorporate these exercises into your day, every day.

Shoulder Shrugs

Aim: To increase respiration and squeeze tension out of shoulders.

Helpful Hints:
- Try saying to yourself "inhaling lifting" as your shoulders go up, and "exhaling dropping" as your shoulders go down. This will help focus your mind away from its stressful antics and get you breathing more deeply.
- Realize that your ribcage goes all the way up to your collarbones. When you drop your shoulders, your ribs are there to rest them on.

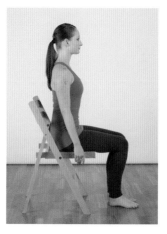 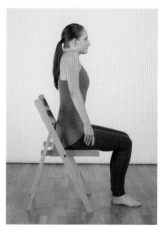

1 Sit comfortably so that your arms can hang down by your sides. Inhale gently and lift your shoulders slowly up into your ears. Keep your mental focus on the co-ordination of your breath with the lifting and dropping of your shoulders.

2 Take as long as the breath takes and see if you can "stretch" your breath as you continue to lift your shoulders higher and higher. Exhale with a soft, open jaw and allow your shoulders to fall back down.

3 Repeat 3 times or until your shoulders feel heavy and relaxed on your ribcage. And yes, that's where your shoulders live—on your ribcage!

Shoulder Squeezes

Aim: To release tension and increase awareness of shoulder position.

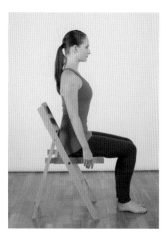 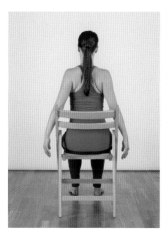

Helpful Hints:
Be aware of your neck as you squeeze your shoulder blades together. Make sure you do not tense it.

1 Sit in the final position of the previous exercise with your shoulders soft and relaxed on your ribcage. Keep weight in your sitbones to make sure that you don't extend your lower back.

2 Inhale and squeeze your shoulder blades together behind you. The squeeze should take your upper back into extension and lift and open your chest. Keep breathing in until you are full, and then with a fast sigh stop squeezing your shoulders and let your chest drop and relax.

3 Repeat 3 times or until your chest feels lifted, open, and relaxed as you breathe normally and your shoulders feel they are resting on the back of your ribs.

41

Shoulder Rolls

Aim: To reposition relaxed shoulders so that they are aligned.

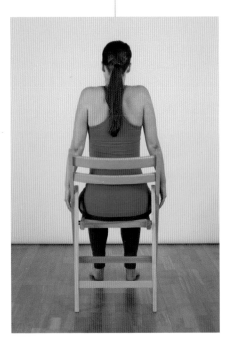 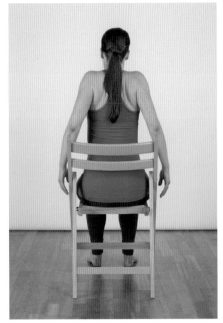

1 Joining the previous two exercises together, inhale as you lift your shoulders as high up as you can, keep your shoulders up and squeeze them together behind you. Think of pulling your head back and up as you squeeze your shoulders together.

2 Exhale quite quickly as if "dumping" the air, and drop your shoulders. Just let go of both. Imagine that you are dropping your shoulder blades back into their rightful place just as you would drop your cell phone in your pocket.

3 Repeat 3 or 4 times.

Chicken

Aim: To counteract the "forward head" that most of us have, which is made so much worse by desk and computer work.

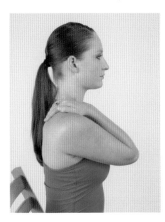
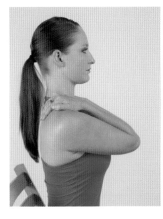

Helpful Hints:
• Hopefully, your head will not need to go as far forward as before.
• Your chest will float up and open as you pull, and you will get taller.

1 Place your hands on your shoulders either side of your neck, palms down with your fingers at the back pointing down. Make sure that your face is looking straight ahead throughout.

2 Keep breathing fluidly as you pull your head up and back, countering with your hands pulling down and forward. Think of the pull being equal and opposite in direction.

3 Hold for 5–8 seconds and release. Don't be surprised if you feel the work between your shoulder blades as you press your head back and up.

Caution:
Many people struggle with a tendency to thrust the head forward, as pictured here. This puts undue strain on the neck and upper back.

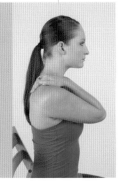

43

Side Neck Stretch

Aim: To release neck and shoulder tension and maintain alignment.

Helpful Hints:
If your shoulders tense with your hands up—simply drop your arms by your sides, being sure to keep your shoulders down and back, and your chest open.

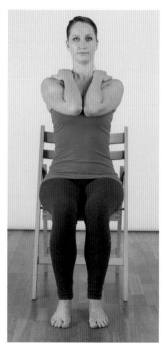
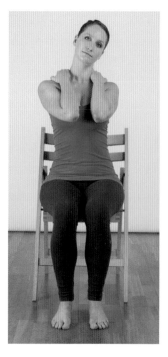

1 Keep your head back in the end position from Chicken (see page 43), with hands still on your shoulders, making sure your arms are heavy, chest open, and shoulders soft and relaxed.

2 Think of lifting your head up off your shoulders and tip your left ear toward your left shoulder.

3 Inhale and raise your head back to center and up again then exhale to the right.

4 Repeat 4—5 times on each side.

Progression:

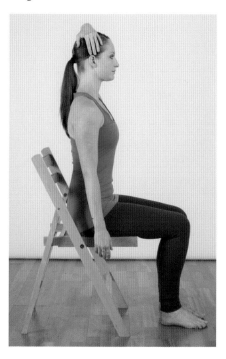

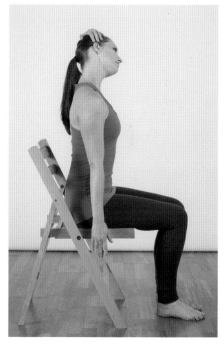

1 If you want more stretch, take your head to the left and place your left hand over your right ear.

2 Inhale and lift your right ear upward into your hand; exhale and increase the stretch. Do not pull on your head. The resistance is gentle.

3 Breathe 2 or 3 times like this and gently release.

4 Repeat to the right.

Helpful Hints:
Make sure that you do not sidebend with your whole body, this is small and focused around your neck/shoulder.

Upper Back Stretch

Aim: To release your midback—this feels especially good down the computer-mouse-arm side of your body.

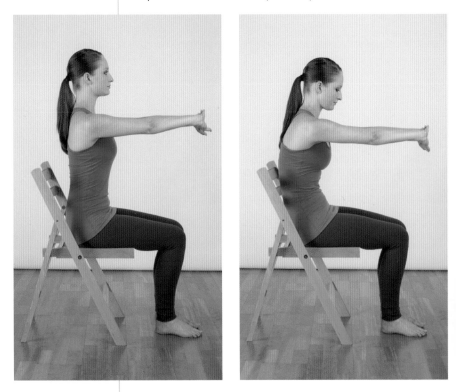

1 Sitting upright, interlace your fingers, turn your palms away from you, and reach your arms out in front of you.

2 Round your back and take a deep breath into your upper back. Exhale and push your hands further forward, increasing the stretch. Inhale deeply as you tilt a little to the right. Exhale to the center. Inhale to the left, exhale to center. Continue this until your sides feel softer and you can breathe more easily.

Kickback Stretch

Aim: The activation and release makes sitting taller easier when you relax in center again. Opens up your chest for fuller breathing.

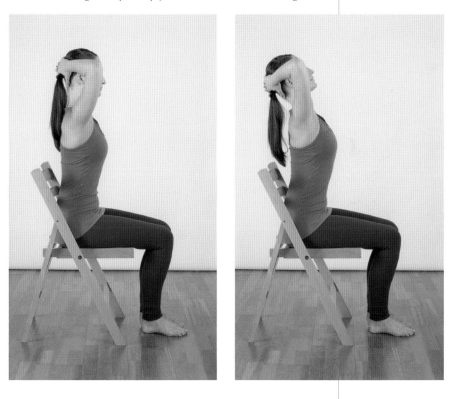

1 Sitting up against the backrest of your chair, interlace your hands behind your head.

2 Inhale and lean back into your hands allowing your back to arch over the top of your chair if you can. Ideally, you will be backbending just below your shoulder blades. Exhale and—without losing your extension—see if you can soften your front lower ribs. Inhale again to reach a little more back and up, and as you exhale to relax your ribs in the front again.

47

Kickback Side Stretch

Aim: To increase lung capacity, open chest, and relax shoulders.

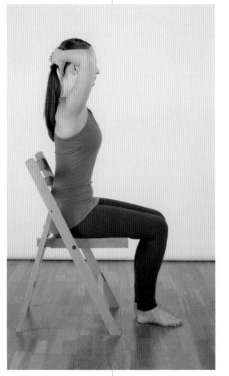 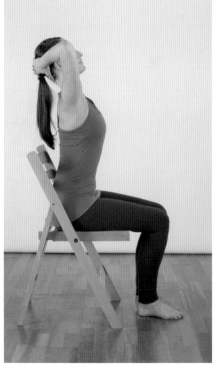

1 Sit in the neutral position with your hands interlaced behind your head.

2 Inhale and lift your chest a little, just like the beginning of the Kickback Stretch.

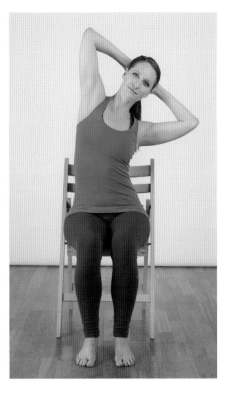
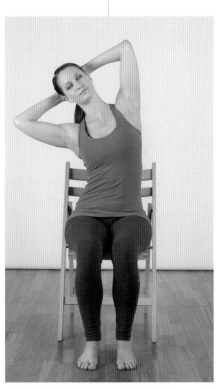

3 Exhale and tip your left elbow diagonally downward to the floor as you lift your right elbow diagonally up to the ceiling. Feel the line of pull from your right elbow all the way to your right hip.

4 Inhale, reach taller and exhale, increasing the bend to the left.

5 Repeat once more and then return to center. Repeat the sequence to the right.

49

Modified Saw

Aim: To defy gravity and its downward pull on your spine, while encouraging the lifting up and creating of space between vertebrae.

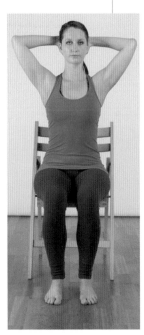 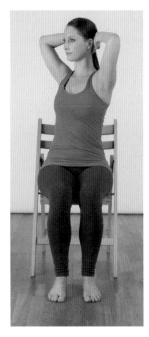 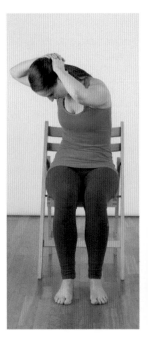

1 Interlace your fingers, and place your hands behind your head.

2 Inhale to drop your sit bones into the chair and float your head up into your hands as you rotate to the right.

3 Exhale and continue to stretch/lift as you curl toward your right hip. Inhale to uncurl your spine and return to center.

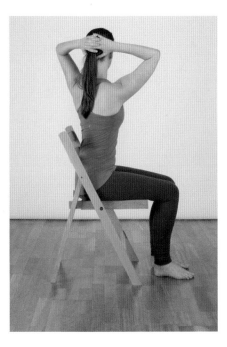 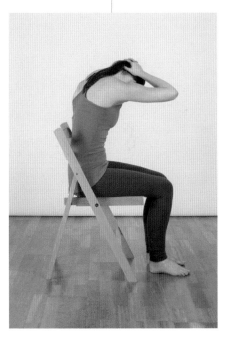

4 Repeat to the left.

5 Repeat each side 3 times.

Helpful Hints:
• As you curl into your hip, keep thinking of reaching your ribs around in the rotation and lifting them up out of your hips.
• You may want to stay in that curl for a breath or 2 before returning to center. Do what feels best.

Thoracic Rotation

Aim: To increase lung capacity and release tension from the whole upper body.

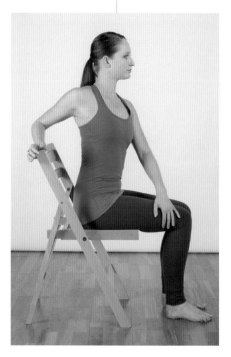 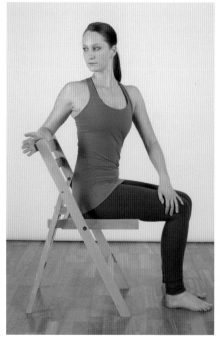

1 Sit in your chair and rotate around to the right to grab the right arm of the chair (or the outside of your right thigh) with your left hand, and reach your right hand to the back of the chair.

2 Inhale into the tightest bit of your back (usually between your shoulder blades and possibly a bit more on the right) growing as tall as possible. Exhale, soften your ribs, and increase the rotation.

3 Repeat 3 times and then come back to center.

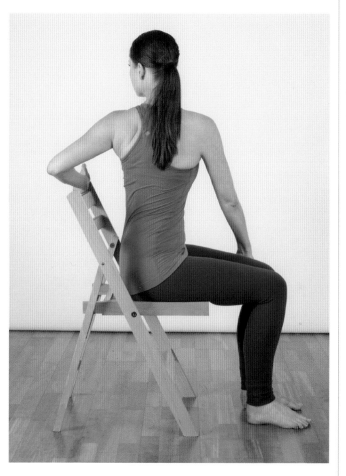

Helpful Hints:
Every time you inhale, think of growing taller. Every time you exhale, gently rotate deeper.

4 Repeat whole sequence to the left.

5 Repeat again on the right and left if you feel you need more!

Forearm Stretches

Aim: To release all the tension stored in your forearms from static mouse and keyboard work.

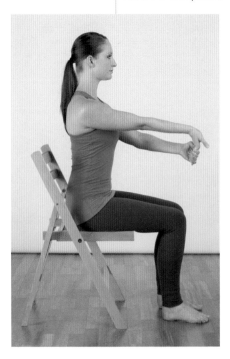 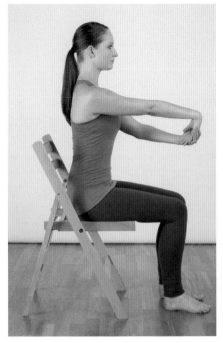

1 Take hold of the fingers of your right hand, turn your right palm away from you with fingers pointing down. Keep pushing your right heel away from you to maintain a straight arm, and gently draw your fingers back toward you to stretch your forearm.

2 Turn your hand around so that your palm is facing you and, again, draw your fingers toward you.

3 Repeat on the left.

54

Puppet Arms

Aim: To release tension and get energy circulating in your arms again.

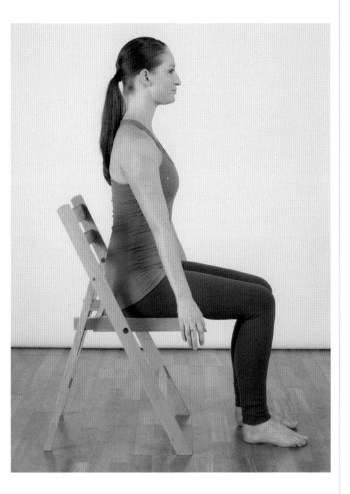

Shake your arms and hands out, feeling any leftover stress falling out, until your arms feel limp, like puppet arms. Don't worry, they will come back even fresher in a moment!

55

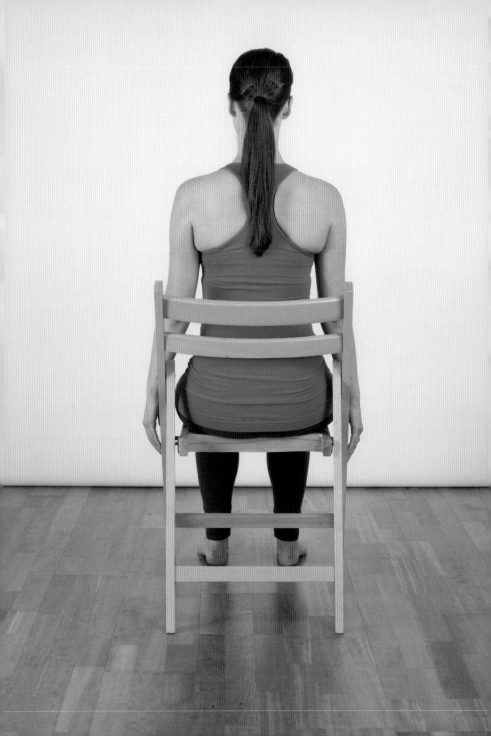

At Your Desk Routine: Lower Back Blues

Bear in mind that even when you're feeling stiff and tight in the lower back, loosening up your shoulders and upper back can help. After all, your upper body is resting on your lower body, and getting a chance to lift it up and off and get your breathing going is invaluable for overall health—and may also be the ticket to really release your lower back. So, if you have time, try both sequences, or alternate them for the best results.

Breathing

Aim: To settle your nervous system and draw a line between the rest of your day and your "me time" with your exercise routine.

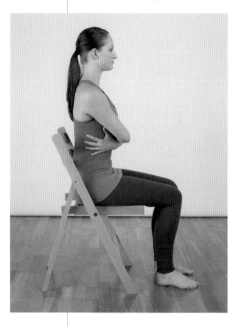

1 Cross your arms at waist height and turn your hands inward to rest on your lower ribs. Hopefully, with your arms folded in this relaxing position, your shoulders will have dropped already.

2 Take a gentle, full breath in, and then with an easy "ha" sound let all the air out. You don't need to force the air, just keep going until the breath tapers out of its own accord.

3 Repeat 3 times.

Helpful Hints:
Simply taking a few minutes to breathe consciously will help to lower your stress levels and prepare you to get the most out your exercise routine.

Progression:
• Take 3 more breaths with the in-breath being the same, but this time, help the breath out with a little effort.
• Notice that your abdominal muscles engage when you breathe out with a little force.
• Keep your belly gently engaged throughout this routine, supporting your spine, and still taking full and deep breaths.

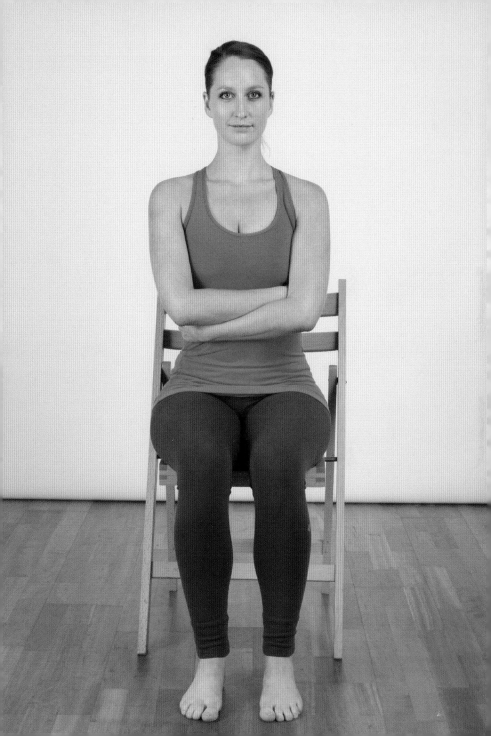

Side Reach

Aim: To open the sides of your torso and encourage deeper breathing.

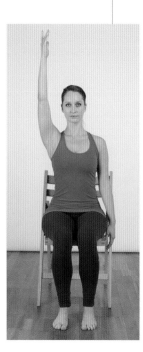 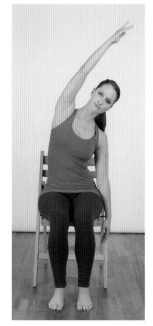 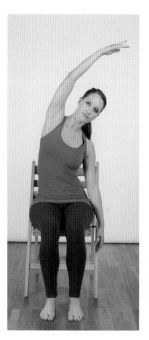

1 Sit in your chair with your arms either resting on the arm rests, or hanging by your sides if you don't have arm rests. Breathe in and reach your right arm up toward the ceiling.

2 Breathe out, continue reaching up and over to the left.

3 Inhale and stay in your side bend, thinking of lifting your right ribs up to the ceiling.

4 Exhale and return your arm to your side. Repeat the sequence with your left arm.

60

Figure Four Stretch

Aim: To release tension in your hips and lower back and get some blood back into your seat.

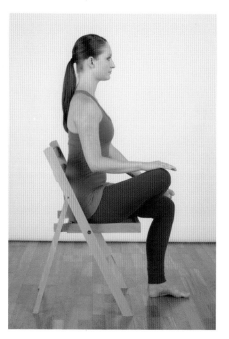
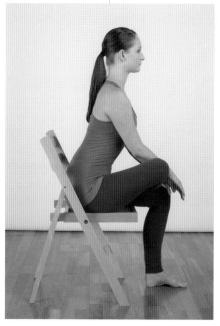

1 Sit with your feet under your knees, hip width apart. Cross your right ankle over your left knee so that your foot is all the way over it. Think of lifting your hips up as much as you can and pitch forward, sticking your bottom right out toward the back of the chair.

2 Lean with your forearms on your right shin and stay here for a few breaths or until your hip feels like it's given in a little!

3 Come out of the stretch and change sides, crossing your left ankle over your right knee. Repeat each side again if needed.

61

Figure Four Rotation Stretch

Aim: To add a side stretch and rotation to the Hip Release on page 150.

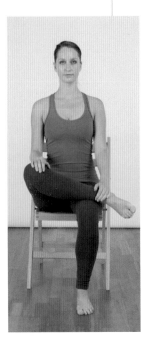 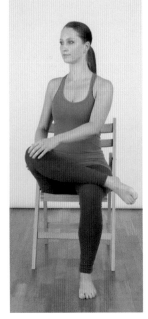 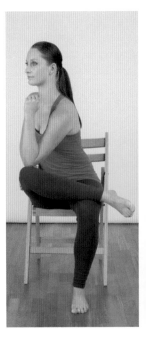

1 Take the same starting position from the previous exercise with your right ankle crossed over your left knee.

2 Brace your right thigh with your right hand and press into it so that you start rotating your torso to the right.

3 Place your left elbow on top of your right knee. Inhale and lengthen your spine as much as possible. Exhale, and press into your knee with both your right hand and left elbow to increase the rotation.

Helpful Hints:
Don't force the movement. Breathing fully and calmly and following the relaxation with every exhale will enable you to increase the stretch.

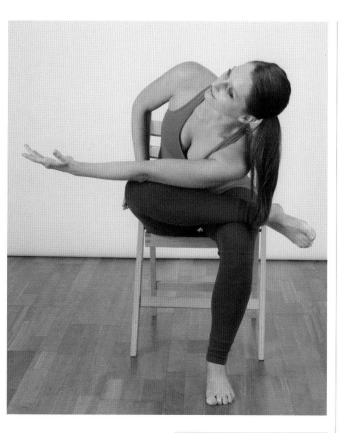

4 Lean your left shoulder toward your ankle as if you were going to lie down on your foot. Take three to four breaths, and on the last exhalation, gently come back to center. Breathe into whichever part of your torso gives the most resistance.

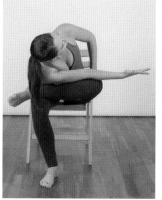

5 Change legs and repeat.

63

Cross Arm Lower Back Release

Aim: To stretch and release tension in the base of your lower back.

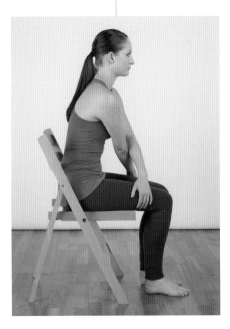 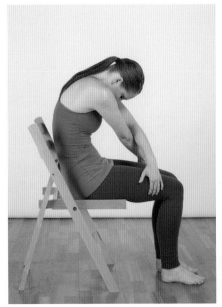

1 Cross your hands over and take hold of the outside of each thigh toward your knees.

2 Squeeze your bottom, pull your belly in, press down with your legs strongly into your hands and curl back. Gaze toward your knees, keeping your neck long and soft. Keep breathing and count slowly to 8.

Lower Back Squeeze

Aim: To increase blood flow and movement in the tissues of the lower back and release tension.

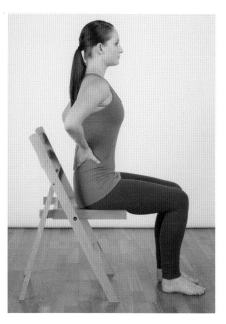 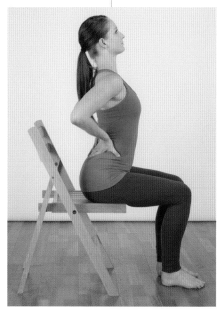

1 Sitting upright, put your hands around the top of your pelvis with your fingertips pointing in and press downward.Continue pressing down with your hands and squeeze the muscles in your lower back making a gentle arch.

2 Lift your chest, and, if you can, take your elbows toward each other. Stay for a count of 4 and gently release. Keep the back of your neck long as you look up, to avoid overextending.

Helpful Hints:
You might like to repeat the last 2 exercises, alternating them for another round or two. They complement each other really well to release stiffness.

65

Hip Hitch

Aim: To wake up and release your sides to make forward and backward bending easier.

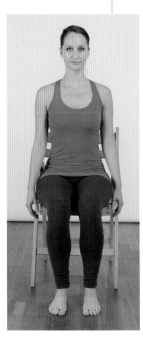
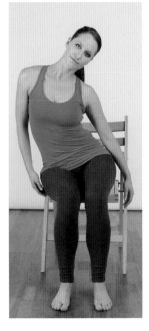

1 Sit at the front of your chair, with your knees bent and feet on the floor under your knees. If you need to, press down into the arms of the chair for support.

2 Exhale and lift your right sit bone off the chair, bending to the right.

3 Inhale and come back to the center.

4 Exhale to lift your left sit bone, bending to the left.

Helpful Hints:
If your chair is on wheels, you can lift your hip and roll your chair a fraction to one side and return it to center.

Progression:

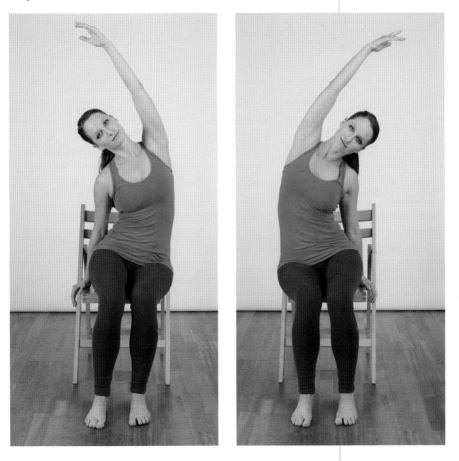

For a deeper stretch, reach your left arm up toward the ceiling as you sidebend to the left, then reach over to your right, stretching through your fingertips. Repeat with the other arm when you are bending to the right.

67

Hamstring Stretch with Arch Curl

Aim: To extend the release of the lower back down the legs and to get the weight off the backs of your legs to allow more blood flow.

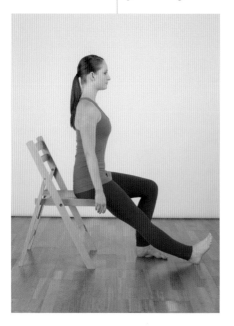
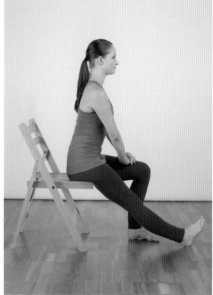

1 Stay forward on the chair and extend your right leg on the floor with your foot flexed.

2 Put the weight of your upper body on your left thigh as you lean forward, sticking your bottom out as much as you can until you get a hamstring stretch on your right leg.

Helpful Hints:
As you move your pelvis relative to your thigh bones, think of your pelvis rolling over and back on the top of your thigh bone and creating more and more space and glide.

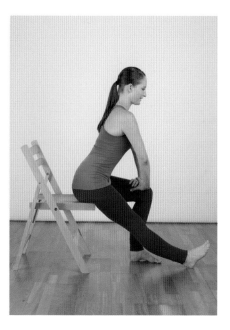
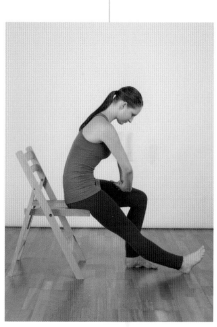

3 Stay forward and gently arch your back.

4 Slowly alternate between an arch and a curl of your lower spine. The stretch will gently increase and ease off as you arch and curl, and over time hopefully you'll be able to increase your forward lean. Rock back and forth about 5–6 times.

5 Repeat on the other side.

69

Cross Legged Upright Spine Twist

Aim: To release tension in the spine and stretch the hips and shoulders.

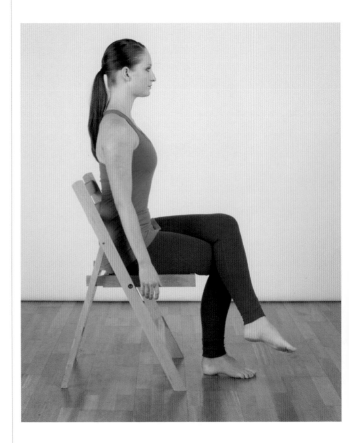

1 Sit in an ordinary cross-legged position with your left leg on top. Inhale gently and let your spine elongate.

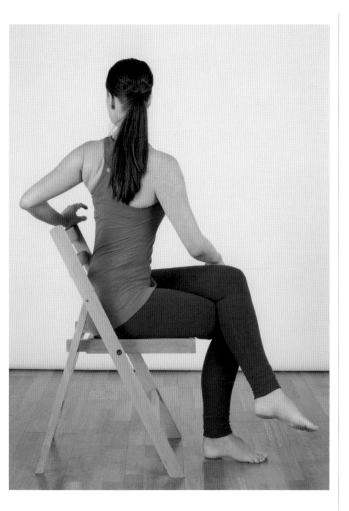

2 Exhale and rotate left using the left arm or back of your chair as leverage. Every inhalation will float you taller, and with every exhalation, soften your ribs, release tension, and increase the rotation.

3 Inhale and rotate back to center, change the cross of your legs and repeat on the right.

71

Seated Hip and Quad Stretch

If you really do not want to get out of your chair and draw attention to yourself, this is a good way to release the hip flexors.

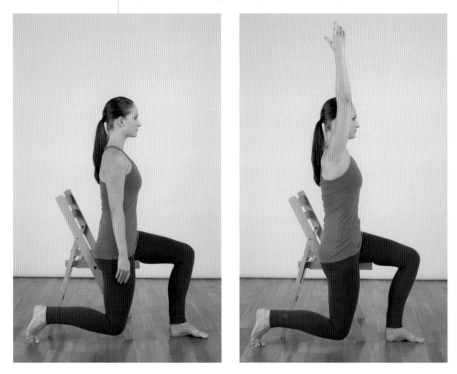

1 Perch on a side of your chair (turn sideways and use the front edge of your seat if your chair has arms). Put your left foot out in front of you, directly under your knee, and tuck your right foot back behind you until your right thigh is vertical. Squeeze your gluteus muscles, especially your right buttock, to press your hips forward. Press into the floor with your left heel and with the ball of your right foot. This position is a great stretch for your hips and the front of your thighs. Lean back slightly to make it harder.

2 Raise your right arm toward the ceiling.

Caution:
Do not do this exercise if your lower back is tense or compressed. Get out of your chair and do the standing versions on pages 62 and 64 instead.

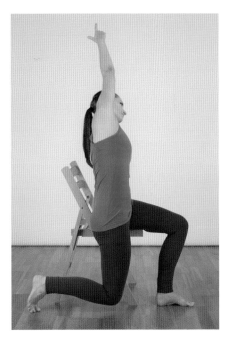
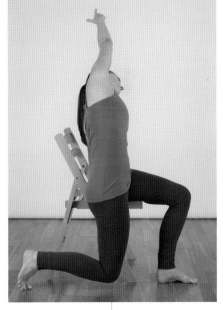

3 Take your right hand over to the left without rotating your hips. You should feel a powerful stretch in your right side.

4 Move to the other side of your chair and assume the reverse position to stretch your other side.

Helpful Hints:
• Keep your abdominal muscles engaged throughout; this is a hip opener, not a back bend.
• Press against the edge of the chair with your thighs to increase the stretch.

73

Standing Hip Stretch

Aim: To open out the front of your hips after being shortened and closed at a desk. To increase breathing.

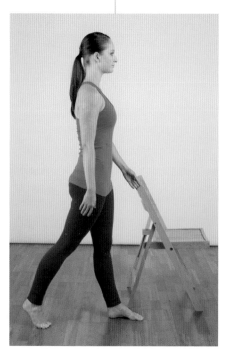
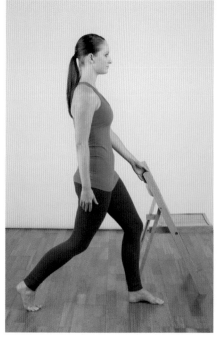

1 Stand with your left leg a long stride in front of your right. Allow your right heel to lift off the floor.

2 Think of lifting your hip bones up as you press your right knee down and back. Squeeze your gluteus muscles, especially your right one to increase the hip stretch.

3 Stay for a couple of deep breaths and change sides.

Progression:

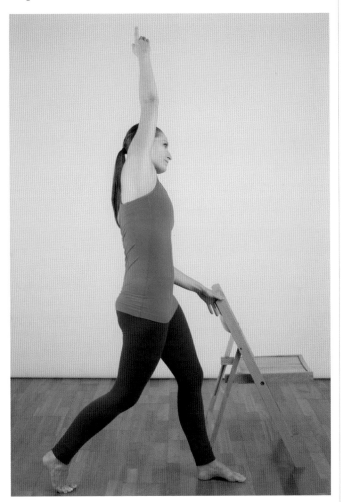

Add a side bend on each side by raising your outside arm up to the ceiling and over your head, reaching with your fingertips.

75

Quad Stretch

Aim: To stretch chronically shortened quadricep muscles caused by long periods of time spent seated.

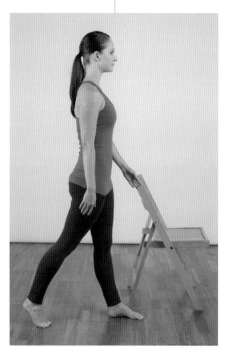 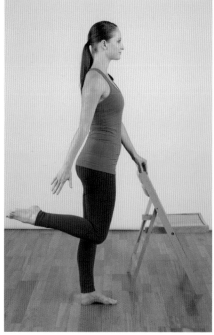

1 Stand beside your chair and hold on to the chair for support.

2 Take hold of the top of your right foot with your right hand, and if you can, with your left hand too.

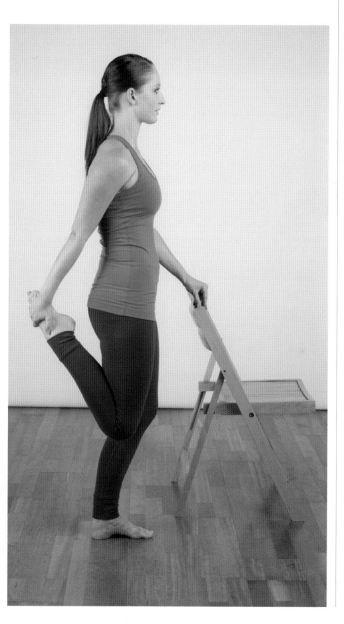

3 Lift your hip bones upward and send your right knee down to the floor. Again, squeezing your gluteus muscles here helps to increase the stretch.

4 Stay for a few deep breaths and change sides.

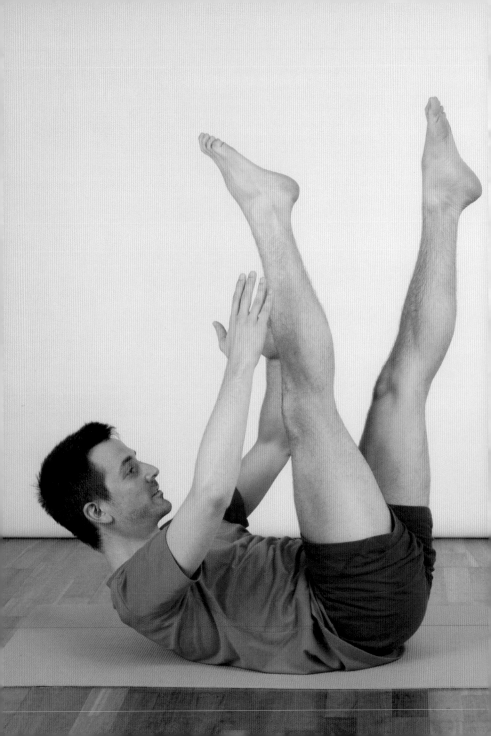

Mat Routine: Revitalize

This routine is short and sweet but has a few challenges in it too. It's good to remember that even when you're short of time, you can still do a few warm-up drills and a few more advanced exercises, then get on with your day. You will notice that a few of these exercises are building blocks toward progressive exercises in the Full Mat Routine that begins on page 158. When you're familiar with the exercises in this section and can perform the full movements or sequences, you might like to incorporate the Full Mat Routine progressions into this routine. This routine will give you a good warm up and a balanced sequence which will be quicker than a full mat routine, but with many of the same challenges.

Roll Down and Shake

Aim: To articulate the spine and release built-up tension from the upper body.

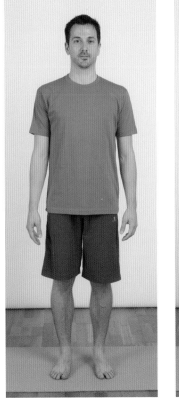

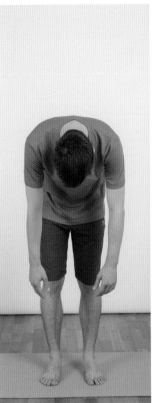

1 Stand with your feet hip-width apart, arms hanging loosely by your sides.

2 Inhale as you nod your head, and as you start to exhale let your chest soften and take you into a roll.

Modification:
• Sit at the front of a chair, separate your legs enough to accommodate your shoulders, and roll down and hang from there.
• Don't worry if your hands are on the floor, just let them flop there.

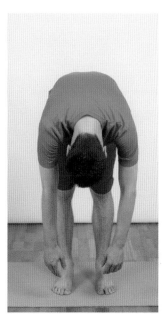 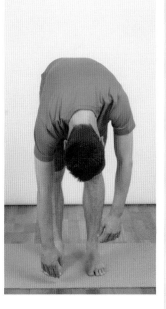

3 Keep your knees soft and when you get as far as you comfortably can, hang there for a few breaths.

4 Wiggle your hips, spine, and head, and shake your arms lightly.

81

Walking Hamstring Stretch

Aim: To release tension in hamstrings, hips, and lower back.

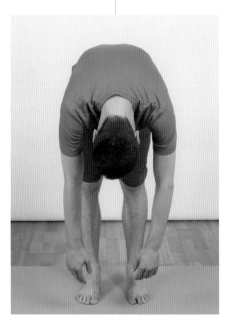 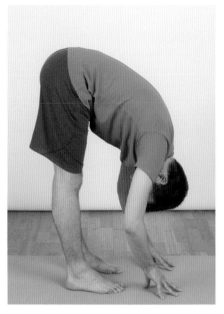

1 Repeat Roll Down (see page 80) and stop again at the bottom.

2 Place your fingertips on the floor, hands under your shoulders.

Modification:
If you cannot reach the floor with your hands, put your hands on a step or seat, or rest them on your shins. Push downwards on your shins for support, not backward into your knees.

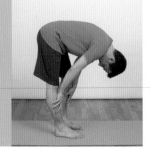

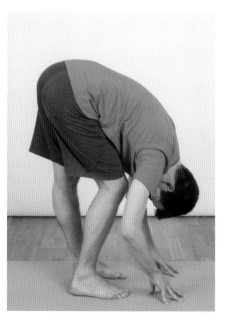 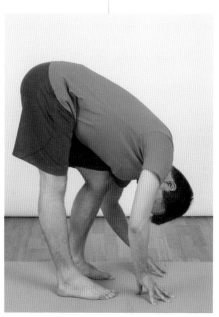

3 Bend your right knee and let your right hip drop. The stretch will increase across your left hip and down that leg.

4 Stay for a few breaths and switch legs. Walk from one leg to the other, breathing easily and fluidly for about 30 seconds.

83

Shoulder Shrugs

Aim: To release neck and shoulder tension.

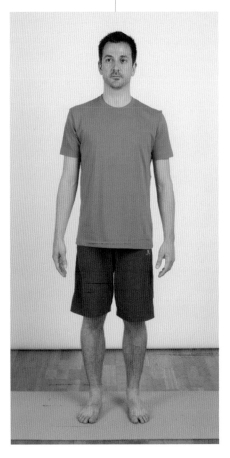

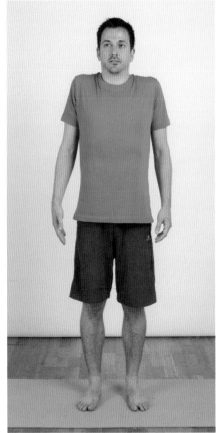

1 Sit or stand with your arms hanging down by your sides.

2 Inhale and shrug your shoulders as high as possible toward your ears.

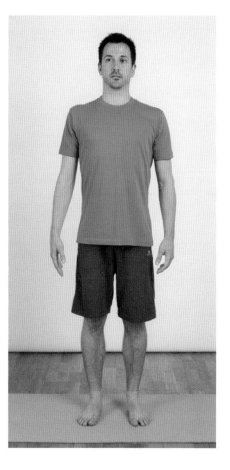

Helpful Hints:
• Keep your chin in as you inhale, and shrug to keep the back of your neck long.
• Keep your chest open as you drop your shoulders, and feel your lower ribs, all the way around, gently soften as if pouring into a funnel.
• Stand tall and keep your spine in neutral with your abdominal muscles drawn in.

3 Exhale with a sigh as you drop your shoulders, and imagine your head floating higher and lighter.

4 Repeat 6 times.

Side Stretch

Aim: To stretch the sides, shoulders, forearms, and wrists.

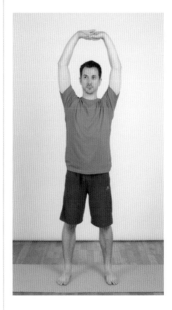 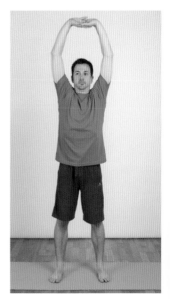

1 Stand with your spine relaxed, your feet just wider than hip-width apart, and knees soft. Interlace your fingers and lift your hands above your head with your palms facing upward.

2 Inhale, allow your arms and shoulders to lift and gently expand your lungs fully in all directions (front, side, back, top, and bottom). Exhale and feel your ribs melt back down.

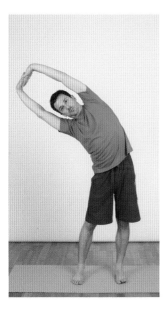 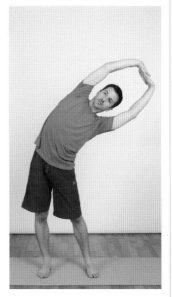

3 Keep your abdominal muscles engaged and, as you inhale, lift up and over to the right. Exhale, return to center, feeling the engagement of your muscles supporting you through the midline.

4 Inhale to reach up and over to the left.

5 Exhale to return to center.

Modification:
If you experience shoulder tension with your hands directly overhead, take your hands slightly in front of you, or bend your elbows to frame your head, and think of lifting through your elbows and armpits.

Squats

Aim: To strengthen buttocks, thighs, and spine, and also to improve posture.

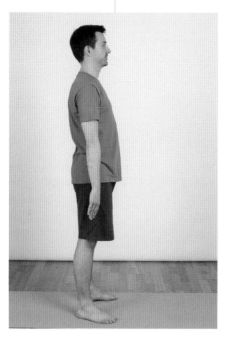 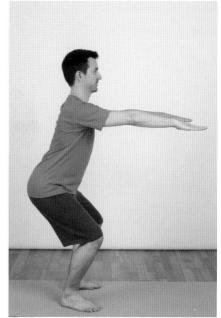

1 Stand with your feet just wider than hip width, hands held in front of your hips. Keep your abdominal muscles drawn in, and maintain a neutral spine throughout the squat.

2 Slowly sit back with your hips as if sitting down in a chair. Allow your spine to flex forward at your hips and take your hands out in front of you to keep your chest up. Ensure your knees do not extend over your toes in the squat.

Caution:
Do not do this exercise if you have an existing back or knee problem unless you have been cleared to do so by a doctor.

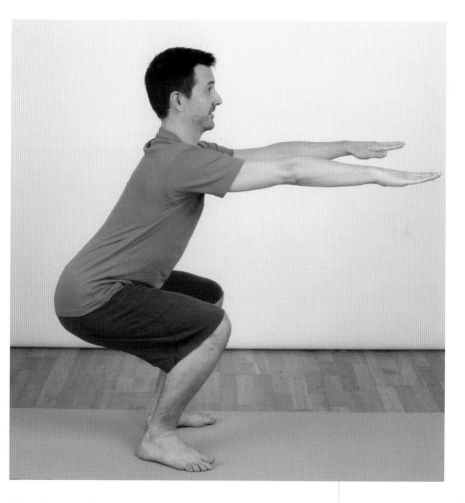

3 Exhale and push your heels into the ground, squeeze your gluteus muscles to press your hips back up to meet your hands in the starting position. If you experience any knee or back discomfort, stop immediately.

4 Repeat 15 times.

Lunges

Aim: To increase strength, power, and co-ordination through lower body to support spine.

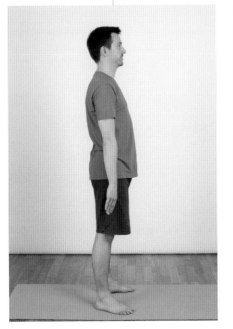 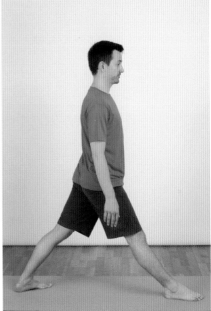

1 Stand with your feet hip-width apart and your arms relaxed by your sides.

2 Inhale and take a long stride forward.

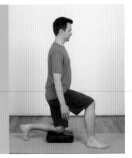

Modifications:
• If you can't get all the way to the floor, put blocks, books, or pillows on the floor for your knee to touch. Slowly reduce the height.
• If the co-ordination is too much and you're wobbling a lot, do all 8 lunges on one side and then swap to the other side.

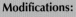

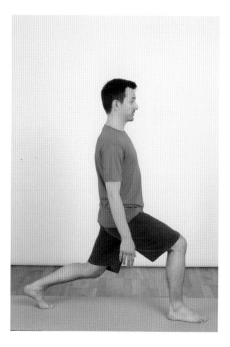 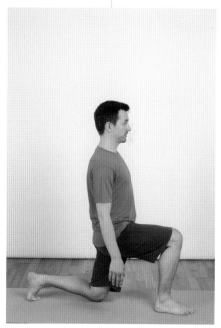

3 As you step forward, bend both knees until your back knee comes down to the floor. Keep your upper body upright throughout—there should be a straight line from your head down to your back knee at the bottom of the lunge.

4 Exhale to press into your front heel and push yourself back to the start position.

5 Repeat with alternate legs for a total of 8 lunges each side.

Kneeling Hamstring Stretch

Aim: To stretch through the chain of muscles in the leg.

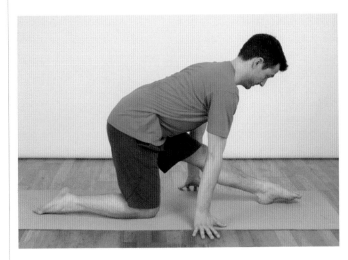

1 Kneel on the floor with one foot outstretched in front of you, one hand on either side of your front foot.

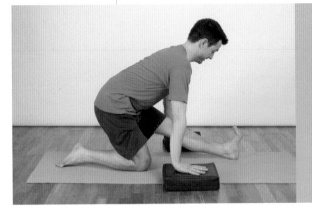

Modification:
If you can't reach the floor, use a prop on one or both sides of your front leg but do not overload your lower back.

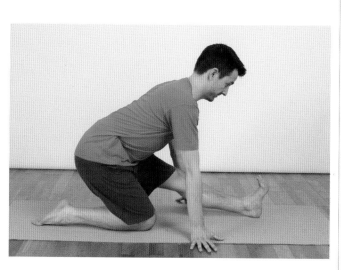

2 Straighten your front leg, press the ball of your foot into the floor, and simultaneously reach your tailbone away from your foot. Flex the front foot to stretch the calf, and alternate between these two positions.

3 Flex and point 8 times on one leg. Move slowly from one position to the next, allowing the body time to ease into the stretch.

4 Repeat on the other side.

Lunge Stretch

Aim: To stretch the front of the hip and release a tight lower back.

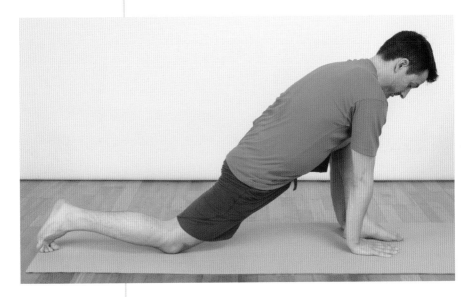

1 Lunge one foot in front of you with one hand either side of your front foot. Rest your back knee on the floor and tuck your toes under. Relax into this position for 2 deep breaths.

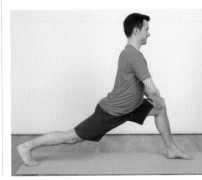

Progression:
If your balance is good, try coming up so that you rest your upper body on your front knee.

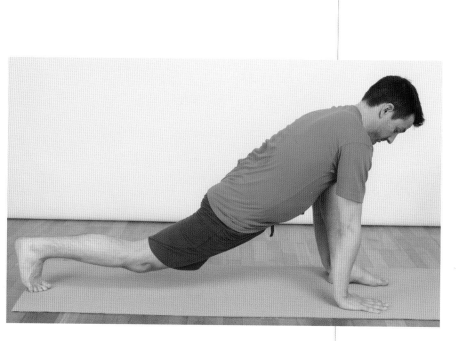

2 Gently lift your back knee off the floor without letting your hips lift. Imagine that your knee lifts because you're reaching your back heel further away from you. Tuck your tailbone under and lift the front of your hips to maximize the stretch.

3 Hold here another 3–5 deep breaths, sinking lower into the stretch with each exhalation if you can.

4 Repeat on the other side.

Elephant

Aim: To stretch back line of the body with abdominal engagement.

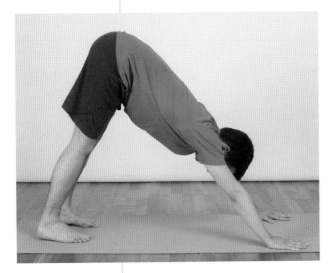

1 Start with hands and feet on the floor, as in an upside down V, with your hips lifting up high toward the ceiling. Keep your shoulders away from your ears and your neck long and relaxed.

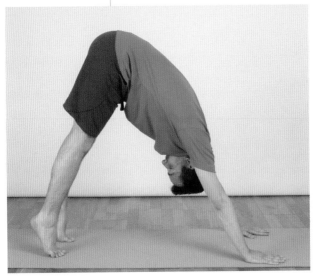

2 Exhale to draw your tail downward to create a C-curl in your spine. Inhale to release your tailbone out behind you to a flat back.

3 Continue to move between these two positions 4–5 times.

Progression:

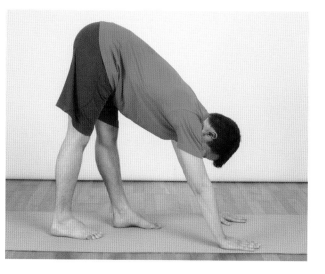

Walk your feet in toward your hands as far as you can with your hands and feet still planted on the floor, and then walk them back out again.

Modification:
• If you can't straighten your legs fully, prop your heels up on a book or block.
• If this is not enough help, bend your knees consciously so that you can focus on the spine movement.

97

Rock 'n' Roll

Aim: To massage the spine, practice maintaining the C-curve and abdominal control.

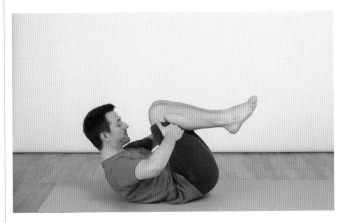

1 Lie on your back, curl up into a C-curve and hug the backs of your knees so your feet are off the floor. Pull your elbows out at the sides to keep your chest open.

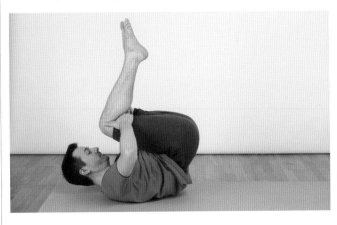

2 Look into your abdominals and inhale to rock backward, but only as far as your waist.

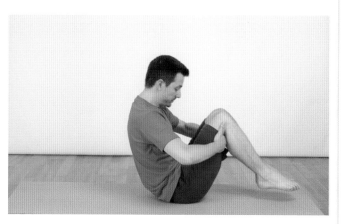

3 Exhale to rock forward onto your sit bones.

4 Continue rocking back and forth, massaging your mid- to lower -back on the floor.

5 Repeat 5–8 times.

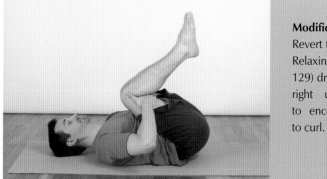

Modification:
Revert to Knee Hugs in the Relaxing Routine (see page 129) drawing your tailbone right up off the floor to encourage your spine to curl.

Single Leg Stretch

Aim: To challenge centerline balance/co-ordination, and increase abdominal control.

Helpful Hints:
Take your leg only as low as you can control your pelvis and maintain your abdominal control.

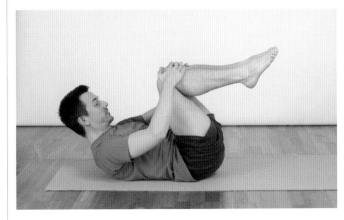

1 Lie on your back with upper body lifted in a C-curve and your legs in tabletop position. Your pelvis must stay relaxed in neutral.

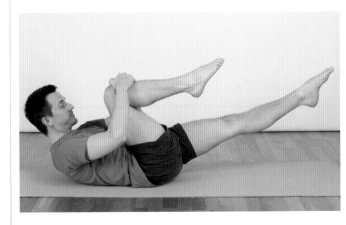

2 Place both hands on your right knee and extend your left leg up toward the ceiling.

100

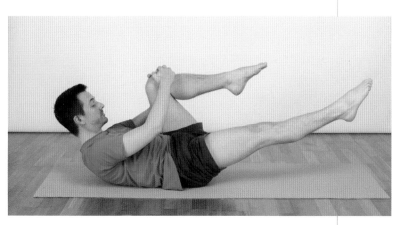

3 Exhale to switch legs, drawing the bent leg deep into your chest for a back release. Don't worry about breathing in—it will happen quite naturally if you concentrate on breathing out.

4 Keep switching legs, exhaling as you hug your knee into your chest.

5 Repeat 10 times, alternating legs.

Progression:
Drop your extended leg a little further away from you for more challenge—keep your pelvis and lower back stable at whatever height you choose.

101

Double Leg Stretch

Aim: To challenge abdominal muscles, stabilization of pelvis, and shoulder girdles, and co-ordination between upper and lower body.

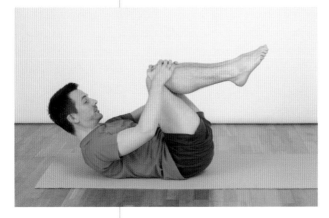

1 Lie on your back with your upper body lifted into a C-curve and your legs in tabletop position. Hold your shins and draw both knees a little toward your chest.

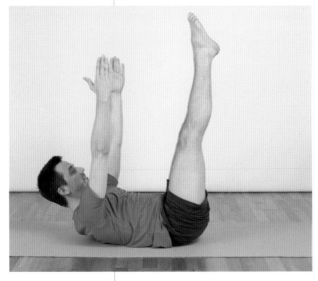

2 Stay in the C-curve, keeping your sacrum anchored into the mat. Inhale and reach both arms and legs up to the ceiling.

3 Exhale and return to the C-curve, grabbing your shins.

4 Repeat 10 times.

Progression:

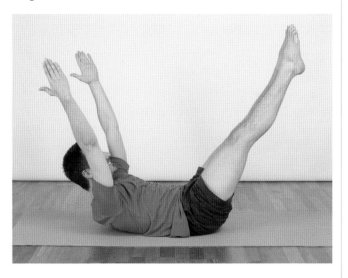

Increase the distance of your arms and legs from the midline without sacrificing your C-curve.

Helpful Hints:
• Breath strongly into the inhale and the exhale to support the movement. This exercise should be strong and punchy.
• Take your arms and legs equal distance away from the midline.

103

Scissors

Aim: To challenge abdominal muscles, with stabilization of pelvis and co-ordination between upper and lower body, and left and right sides.

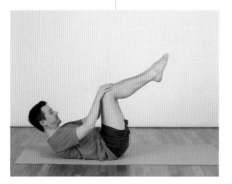

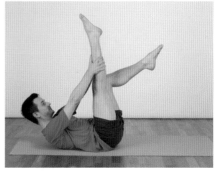

1 Lie on your back with your upper body lifted into a C-curve and your legs in tabletop. One hand resting on each knee.

2 Extend your right leg toward the ceiling and take both hands around your calf—or if you can't reach it, your thigh.

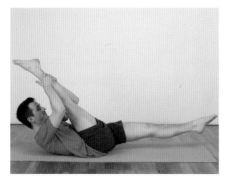

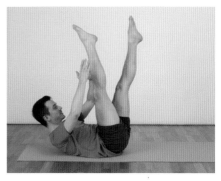

3 Exhale and draw your right leg in toward you, pulse it toward you again.

4 Inhale lightly as you change legs.

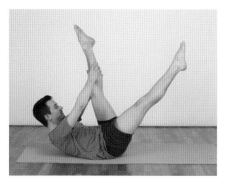

5 Exhale to grab and pulse your left leg in toward you. Alternate 10 times.

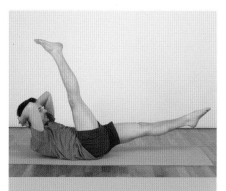

Progression:
Interlace your hands behind your head and keep your legs moving.

Tic Toc

Aim: To strengthen abdominal muscles and create control through upper body stability.

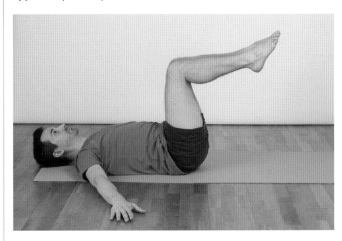

1 Lie on your back with your legs in tabletop position and your arms outstretched by your sides.

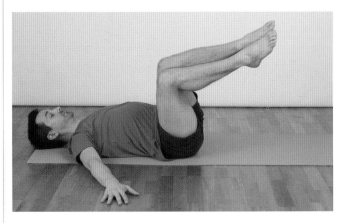

2 Inhale and send your legs only as far to the right as you can without your left shoulder coming off the floor. Exhale to return to center.

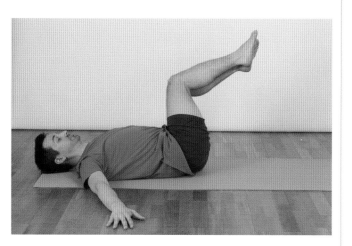

3 Inhale to go to the left. Exhale to center.

4 Repeat 5 times to each side.

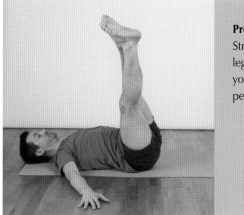

Progression: Straighten your legs and Tic Toc your legs like a pendulum.

Glute Press with Transfers

Aim: To further challenge glute and leg strength, and achieve abdominal control.

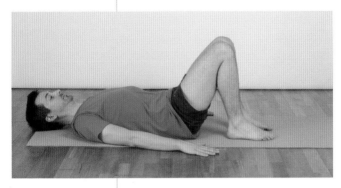

1 Lie on your back with your knees bent and your feet flat on the floor, arms resting by your sides.

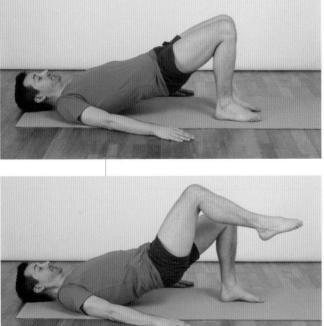

2 As you exhale, squeeze your gluteus muscles and lift your hips into the air. Inhale and hold.

3 Exhale and lift one foot off the floor, taking care not to let the hip on that side drop. Inhale and place the foot down.

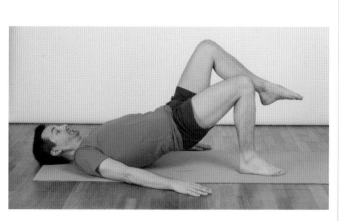

4 Exhale, and lift the other foot (again watch the hip). Inhale and replace the foot.

5 Exhale hold and reassert the squeeze on your gluteus muscles before you inhale and release your torso back to the ground.

6 Repeat this 6 times, alternating the starting leg each time.

Helpful Hints:
• Keep pressing down into the heel of the supporting leg to activate your hamstring and gluteus muscle.
• Don't let your back arch or hip drop as you lift your leg.

Breast Stroke Preparation

Aim: To strengthen spinal extensors and shoulder stability.

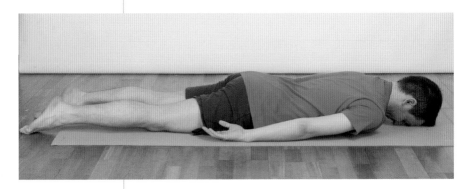

1 Lie on your stomach with your arms long by your sides and your forehead on the mat. Breathe in, and as you breathe out engage your abdominal muscles to prepare

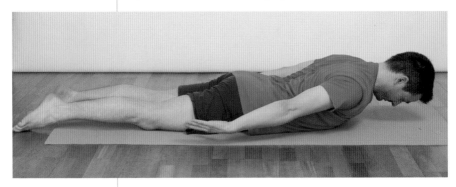

2 As you breathe in, lift your head and upper back without shortening or compressing your lower back. Stay for a count of 3, and release down. Repeat 5 times.

Be mindful of your lower back during this movement. Stop if it feels compressed at all.

Progression:

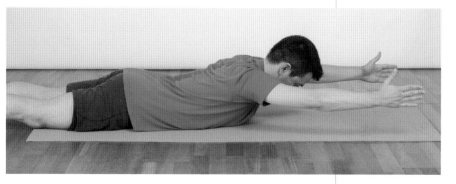

1 While your torso is lifted, bring the arms forward until they extend fully in front of you.

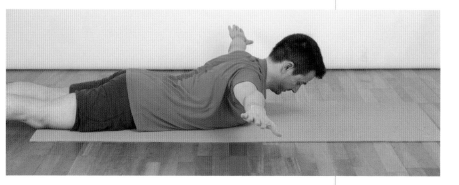

2 Turn palms to face outward and bring your arms fully out to your sides, then back in to your sides. Repeat 5 times as a fluid motion.

111

Leg and Arm Extensions (Swimming Preparation)

Aim: Challenge of pelvis and shoulder stability and freedom of movement for arms and legs. Increase endurance for spinal extensors.

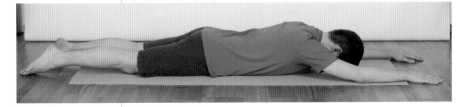

1 Lie on your stomach with your arms extended above your head and your forehead on the mat.

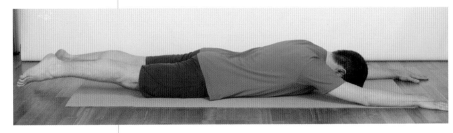

2 As you breathe out, feel your midline naturally engage. Maintain that feeling as you inhale to lift your legs off the mat.

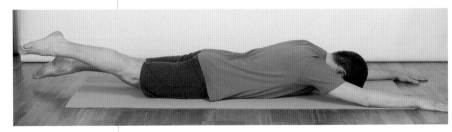

3 Alternately lift one leg more than the other, and as you switch legs, call that one "kick." Exhale as you kick your legs, switching 5 times. Inhale, continue kicking for 5 beats.

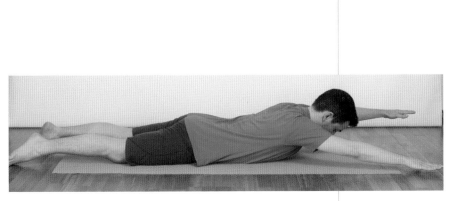

5 Rest your legs down. Inhale to extend your arms off the mat. Alternately lift one arm more than the other, and as you switch arms, call that one "switch".

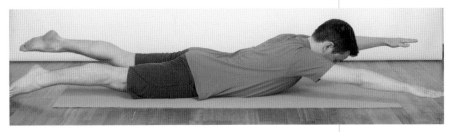

6 Exhale, as you switch your legs 5 times. Inhale continue switching for 5 beats.

This is another exercise which can compress the lower back. If your back feels at all uncomfortable, engage your abdominal muscles more strongly and minimize your lifting. If discomfort persists, stop the exercise.

Front Support

Aim: To strengthen shoulders, torso alignment, and whole body co-ordination (face down).

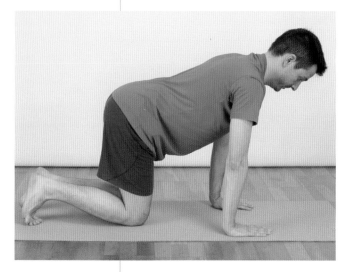

1 Start on your hands and knees, with your toes tucked under. The closer your feet are together, the more challenging the movement—so choose your distance.

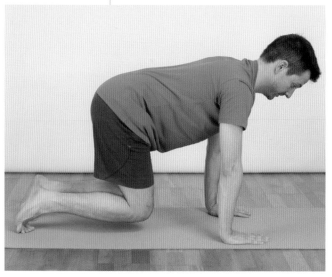

2 Push into your hands and the balls of your feet to lift your knees off the mat. Press the floor strongly away from you so that your shoulder blades hug your ribcage rather than "winging out."

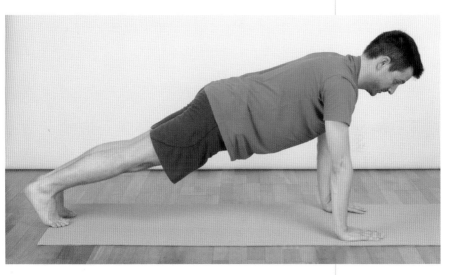

3 Step back into a plank position with your hands underneath your shoulders and your legs outstretched, toes tucked under.

4 Hold for 30 seconds, lower yourself down to the floor to rest and take 2 deep slow breaths, then go back up for another 30 seconds. Keep your midline strong—no sagging in the middle!

Modification:
• Start on all fours with your shoulders over your hands and hips over your knees, tuck your toes under.
• Breathe in and, engaging your abdominals, lift your knees off the floor and hold, breathing naturally for a count of 10.

115

Side Support

Aim: To strengthen shoulders, torso alignment, and full body co-ordination.

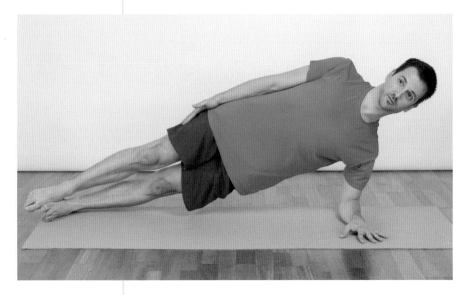

1 Lie on your side with your legs outstretched, propped up on your elbow with your forearm on the ground at 90 degrees to your body.

2 Breathe in, and as you breathe out engage your abdominal muscles, press down into your forearm, and lift your hips off the floor. Hold for 30 seconds, come down and take 2 deep slow breaths—then go back up for another 30 seconds.

3 Change sides and repeat.

Progression:

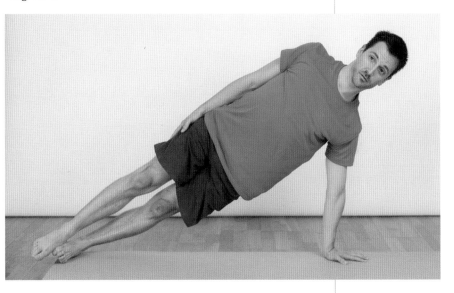

Balance on your hand instead of your elbow.

Modification:
Bend your bottom knee and use it as leverage to keep you up.

117

Back Support

Aim: To strengthen shoulders, torso alignment, abdomnial muscles, and whole body co-ordination.

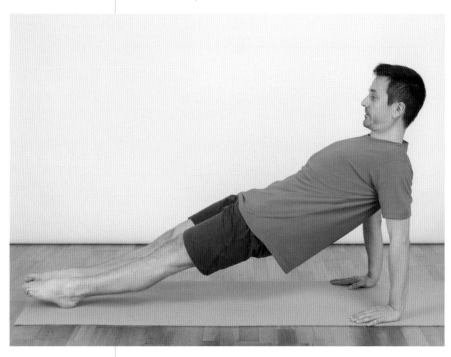

1 Sit on your mat with legs outstretched in front of you and hands behind you, shoulder-width apart, fingers facing forward.

2 Take a breath in and as you breathe out, press your pelvis into the air to create a straight line from your feet through your hips to your head.

3 Stay looking forward as you hold for 30 seconds. Slowly lower your pelvis down and take two breaths before repeating a 30 second hold.

Modification:

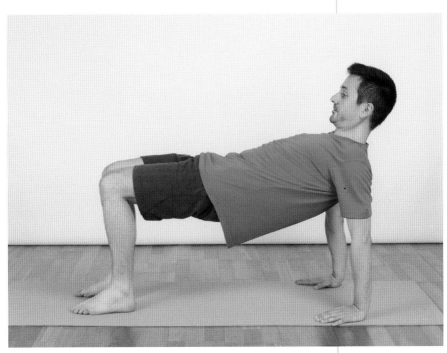

Keep your feet flat on the floor and bend your knees to lift your hips.
The closer in your feet are the easier—so don't cheat too much!

Mermaid

Aim: To strengthen and lengthen the sides of the torso and support breathing.

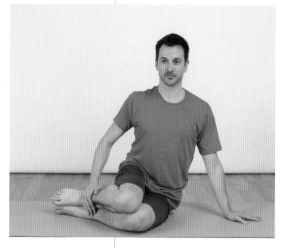

1 Sitting on your left hip, tuck your legs to your right side so that the outside of your left leg is resting on the ground and your right leg is stacked on top.

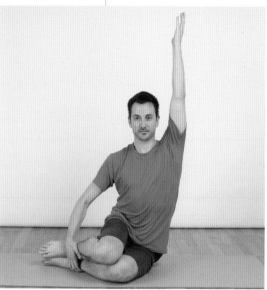

2 Inhale to reach your left hand up toward the ceiling.

3 Exhaling, reach your left hand over to your right, leaning into a side bend. You should feel this stretch all along your left side. Enjoy for a few breaths, then drop your left hand to the start postion on an exhale.

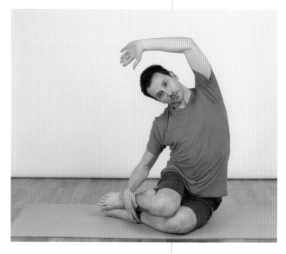

4 Come down onto your left elbow and inhale to lift your right arm up and over to your left, stretching your right side.

5 Exhale to return to your starting position and repeat the sequence.

6 Change sides and repeat twice.

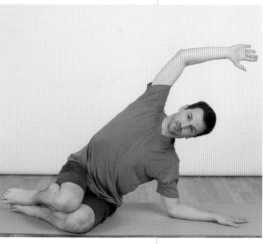

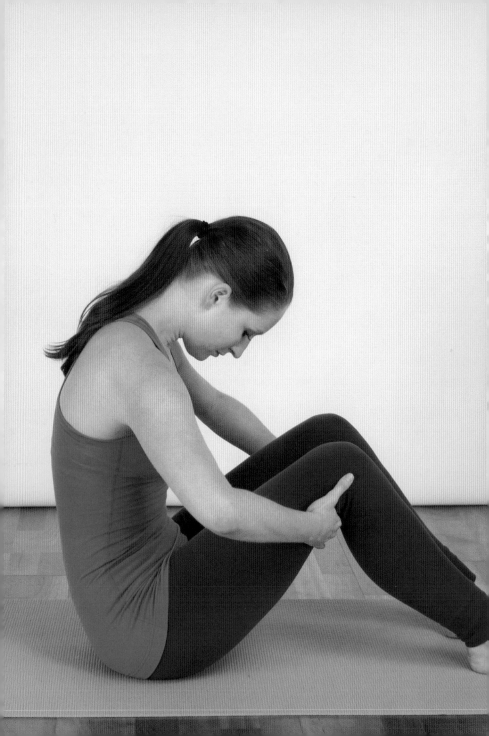

Mat Routine: Relax

The Relax routine is perfect for when your nervous system is wound up and you need to take time out to become centered again. It's very tempting to do nothing when you're exhausted, but gentle mobilizing movements will increase energy flow in your body and not take too much time. This is perfect for rebalancing. It's also important to stay in the habit of doing some exercise—otherwise, when you do have the energy, you may not have the motivation. Why not try the Relax routine fairly close to bedtime? You might even drift off to sleep in the middle of it!

Hip Rolls

Aim: To increase mobility throughout your spine and hips.

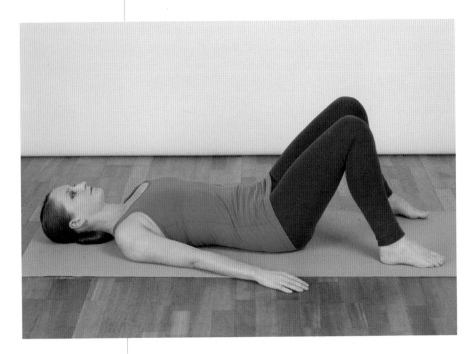

1 Lie on your back with your knees bent, feet flat on the floor wider than your hips, and arms comfortably out to the sides.

Helpful Hints:
• Make your legs as heavy and passive as possible.
• Your bottom knee should relax onto the floor, your top knee will reach away from you so that the stretch is down the front of that thigh.
• The stretch may extend through to your hip and lower back, and even up to shoulder height.

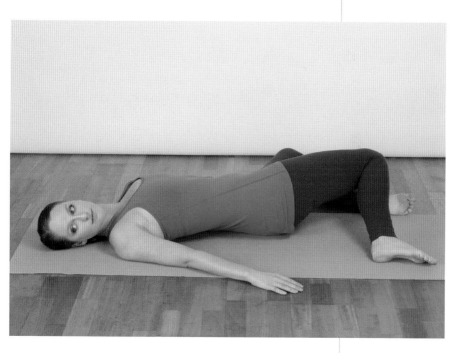

2 Allow your knees to fall gently to the left. Roll your head to the right at the same time.

3 Return to center.

4 Repeat on the other side, so knees go to the right, head rolls to the left. Return to center and repeat 3 times on each side.

Around the World

Aim: To achieve a full body release and increase respiration.

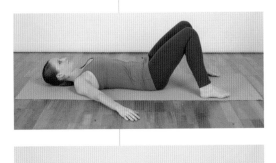

1 Lie on your back with your knees bent, feet flat on the floor wider than your hips, and arms comfortably out to the sides.

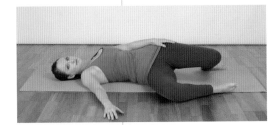

2 Allow your knees to fall to the right.

3 Draw your left hand down past your left hip, across to your right knee.

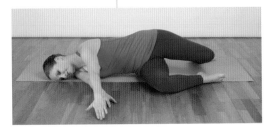

4 As you roll onto your right-hand side, reach your arm over your head.

5 Imagine yourself from above and draw the biggest horizontal circle you possibly can with your moving hand.

6 Continue to circle your arm until it comes to rest in its starting position.

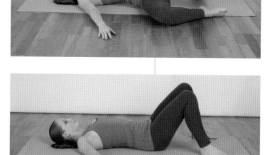

7 Return your knees to center and continue letting them fall over to the left. Circle your right arm past your right hip, over toward your left knee and overhead; then rest it back by your side.

8 Draw two full alternate circles in each direction.

Knee Hugs

Aim: To lengthen and release lower back and hips.

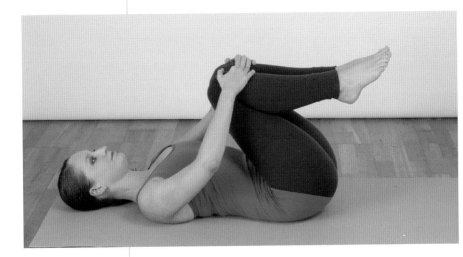

1 Lie on your back with your knees drawn up toward your chest.

Helpful Hints:
• Imagine the air reaching all the way down to your tailbone and lower belly as you breathe in. Feel the weight of your tailbone resting on the floor (if you can.)
• Don't let your shoulders tense to squeeze your knees in. Use the strength of your arms and be patient. You will increase your flexibility more by working with your breathing than by forcing things.

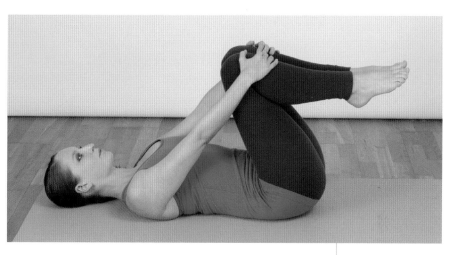

2 As you inhale, float your knees away from your chest until your arms are straight.

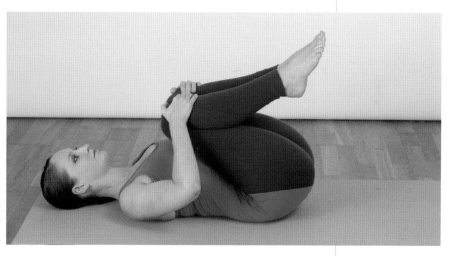

3 Exhale and draw your knees closer to your chest—think of your knees following the breath out of your body.

4 Repeat 10 times.

129

Knee Circles

Aim: To release lower back and relax whole body.

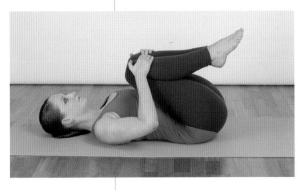

1 Hug your knees in toward your chest. with a hand on each knee

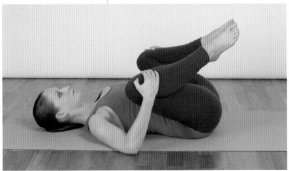

2 Separate your knees and inhale as you circle them away from you, back together, and in to your belly again.

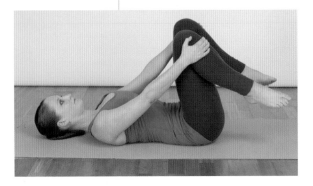

3 Take 5 circles in this direction, then change direction for 5 more circles. Feel as if you are stirring your thigh bones in your hip sockets. Aim for a gliding sensation.

The Fan

Aim: To stabilize pelvis and enable free movement of the thigh in the hip.

1 Lie on your back, knees bent, feet flat on the floor and side by side.

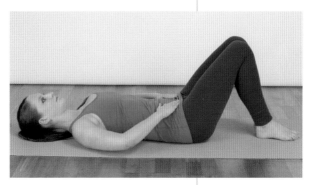

2 Allow your right knee to fall out to the right without any movement of your other leg or of your pelvis. When the stability is challenged, return to center.

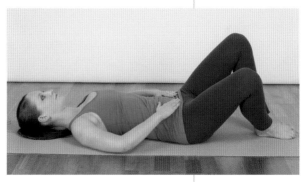

Helpful Hints:
- Breathe fluidly throughout the exercise.
- This is one where the smallest movements count.
- Your task is to keep your pelvis stable without getting tense in your neck, shoulders, or jaw.

131

Pelvic Press and Roll

Aim: To strengthen and tone buttocks and backs of thighs.

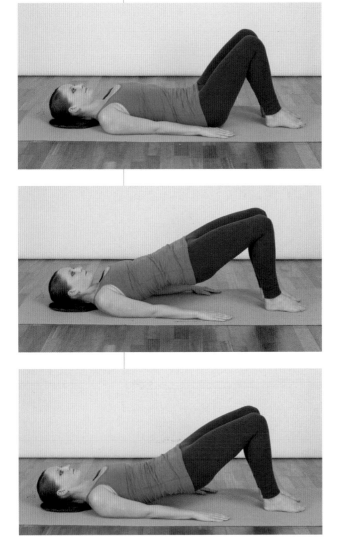

1 Lie on your back with your knees bent and feet flat on the floor, arms resting by your sides.

2 As you inhale, press down into your feet—especially your heels—and lift your hips up until they are in line with your chest and knees.

3 Exhale and roll your spine gradually back down to the floor.

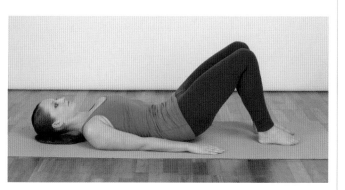

4 Repeat 3 times—when you're ready to move on, add arms (see page 134).

Variation:
Start with your feet on a chair to give you more height, but take care not to rest weight any higher than your shoulders when you press up.

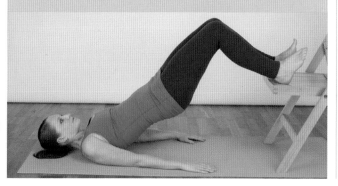

133

Pelvic Press and Roll with Arms

Aim: Adding arm movements makes the Pelvic Press and Roll a much more difficult exercise.

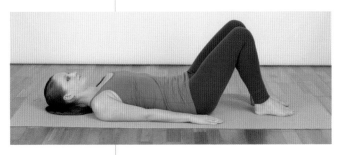

1 Lie on your back with your knees bent and feet flat on the floor, arms resting by your sides.

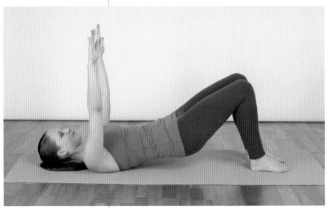

2 Lifting your pelvis, as for the Pelvic Press and Roll (see page 132), take your arms over your head to a diagonal behind you. Keep your abdominals contracted and use your core strength.

Helpful Hints:
This exercise is not a tilt on the way up where you would roll your spine off the floor. Your back comes up in one clean movement and then rolls back down. This should be a little easier to manage than tilting in both directions, and should give you a lovely stretch to boot. Watch that your back doesn't arch at the top. You should remain stable through your pelvis and lower back.

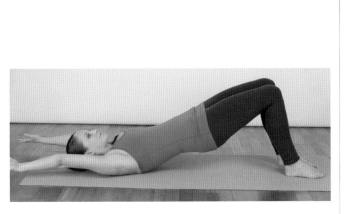

3 As you roll back down through your spine reach away with your hands and feel the stretch all the way down your back.

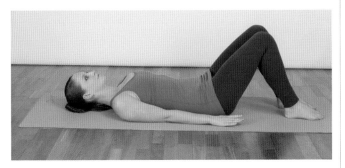

4 Place your arms by your sides. Repeat 3 times.

Half Roll Down

Aim: To increase spinal mobility, length, and control. To stretch lower back.

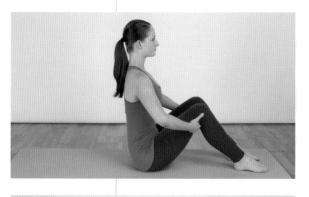

1 Sit with your knees bent, feet flat on the floor, hip width apart, and grasp the back of your thighs just above your knees.

2 Lean back until you have a little space at the front of your hips and then begin rolling your pelvis back until first your sacrum, and ultimately your waist, comes to the floor.

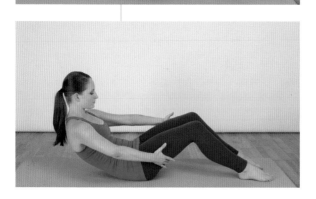

3 Keep breathing naturally. Actively use the resistance of your arms to help your spine articulate and keep you from simply leaning back onto the floor.

4 Pause when you can go no further without straightening your back ,and inhale.

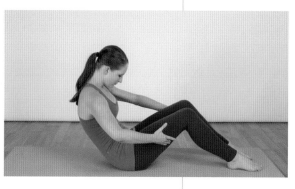

5 Exhale to curl forward again and reach your nose to your knees.

6 Inhale to elongate your spine to the start position and repeat a total of 5 times.

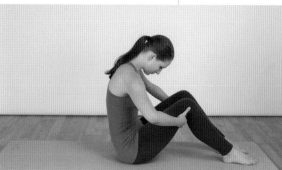

Clam

Aim: To increase control and strength in external rotation of thigh, and challenge stability of pelvis.

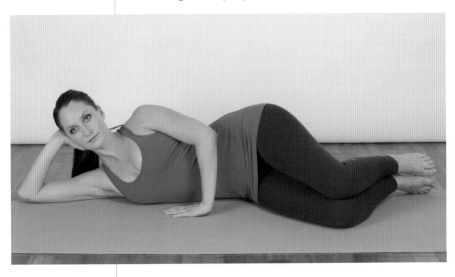

1 Lie on your right-hand side with your knees bent, and your hips, knees and ankles stacked on top of one another.

Helpful Hints:
• Your top hip will want to roll back to assist the movement of your leg. Think instead of leaning your top hipbone into something heavy as you lift your knee. You'll feel the increase in resistance.
• Do this, and the next two exercises as a group—all three on one side, and then roll over and do all three on the other side.

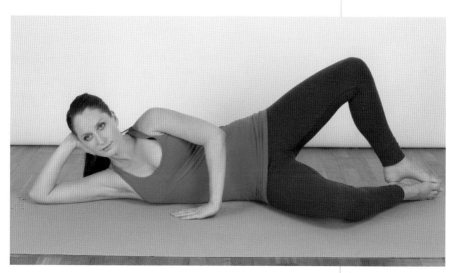

2 Exhale, draw your midline in, and lift your left knee as high as you can without moving your pelvis.

3 Inhale and return your top knee to your bottom knee. Repeat 10 times.

Single Leg Lift

Aim: To strengthen the sides of the hips and torso.

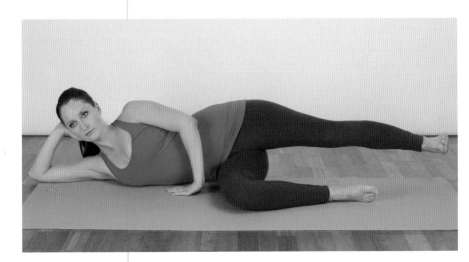

1 Lie on your right hand side with your bottom leg bent and your top leg outstretched.

2 Inhale, and as you exhale, lift your top leg off the floor.

3 Inhale to lower your leg.

4 Repeat 8 times.

Helpful Hints:
- Keep your hips stacked one on top of the other.
- Keep reaching your legs out away from you.
- Keep your neck and head relaxed.

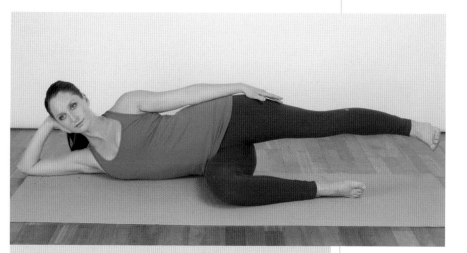

Progression:
To make this exercise more difficult, place your left hand on your hip. You are now anchoring your body position with your abdominal muscles. Keep them engaged throughout the movement.

141

Double Leg Lift

Aim: To strengthen the sides of hips and torso and challenge balance.

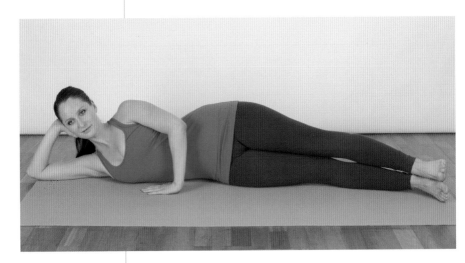

1 Lie on your right-hand side with both legs outstretched, your feet just a little in front of your hips.

Helpful Hints:
- Keep your hips stacked one on top of the other.
- Keep reaching your legs out away from you.
- Keep your neck and head relaxed.

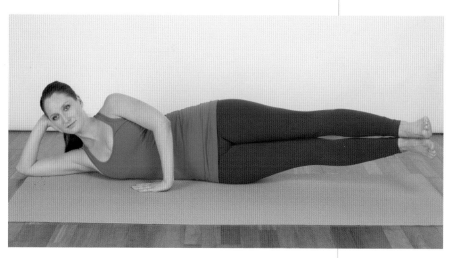

2 Inhale, and as you exhale, lift both legs off the floor.

3 Inhale to lower your legs down.

4 Repeat 8 times.

5 Change sides and do the set of three exercises: Clam, Single Leg Lift, and Double Leg Lift.

143

Superman

Aim: To challenge balance and gently strengthen extensors of the body.

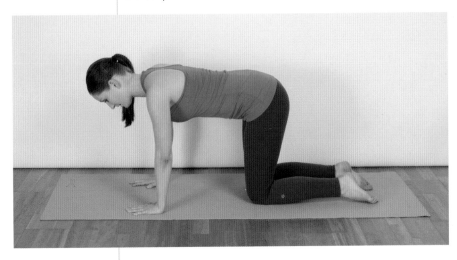

1 Start on all fours with hands under shoulders and knees under hips.

Modification:
Keep your reaching hand and foot on the floor if your balance, energy, or stability do not allow for lifting.

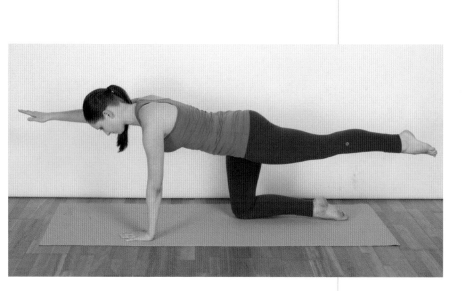

2 Inhale and extend your right arm and left leg away from you and lift them to be perpendicular to the floor.

3 Hold for a count of 3, exhale, then bring your limbs down onto the mat in a controlled way.

4 Inhale and take your left arm and right leg away from you and lift until they are horizontal.

5 Hold for a count of 3, exhale, then bring your limbs down onto the mat in a controlled way.

Prayer Stretch

Aim: To stretch chest and thoracic spine and increase respiration.

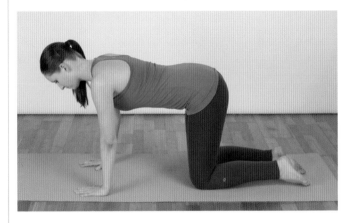

1 Start on all fours with hands directly under shoulders and knees hip width apart.

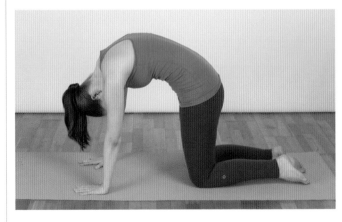

2 Press down into your hands, rounding your back and dropping your head. This is the Cat Stretch (see page 161).

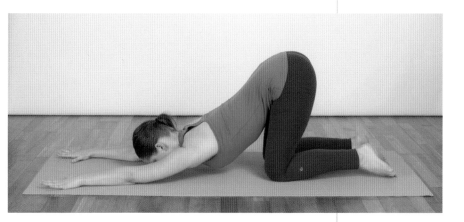

3 Slide your hands forward so your arms are fully extended, while pulling your hips back and up, allowing your chest to reach down and forward. This should feel like a slight back bend.

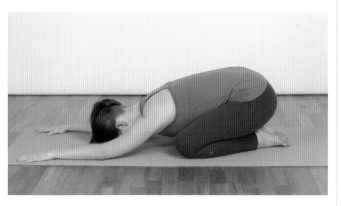

4 Finally, sink back onto your heels, relax the arms, and let your forehad touch the ground. Child's Pose allows your spine to relax for a few moments after the bending and flexing of Prayer Stretch. Feel space opening up between your vertebrae.

147

Thread Needle Stretch

Aim: To rotate the spine and release shoulders and hips.

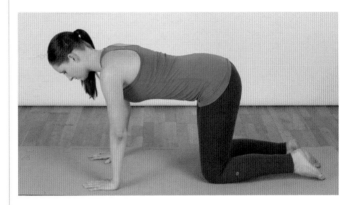

1 Kneel on all fours with hands under your shoulders and knees under your hips.

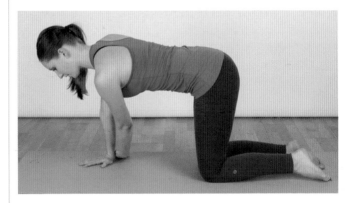

2 Take your left hand off the floor and place it behind your right wrist.

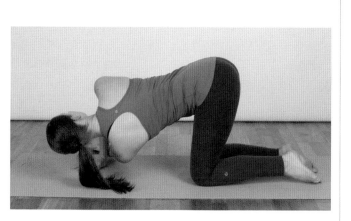

3 Breathe in, and as you breathe out reach diagonally up and out to the right as far as you can so that your chest is lifted and your spine rotates.

4 Breathe in to press down into your right hand and come back to center.

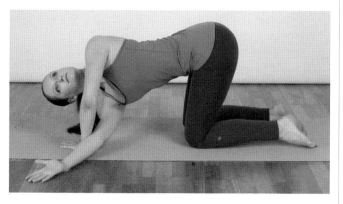

5 Change sides and repeat 4 times.

149

Hip Release

Aim: To release the hips and groin.

Helpful Hints:
• Try to keep your hips even. Reach your back foot as far away from you as possible and roll that hip toward the front foot.
• Relax your spine over your leg and try to let go of your body weight.

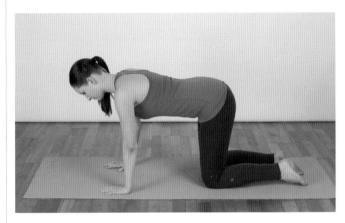

1 Begin on all fours with hands under shoulders and knees under hips.

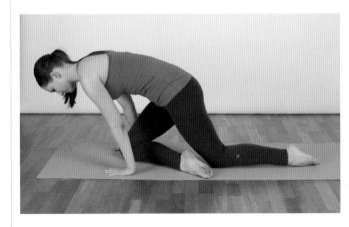

2 Bring your right knee up between your hands and take your right foot as far over to the left as is comfortable.

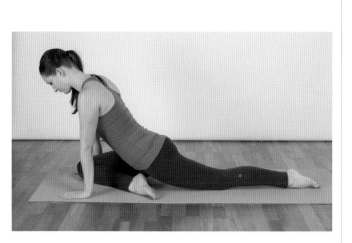

3 Slide your left leg back behind you until you are lying over your right leg and you have a stretch in your right hip and inner thigh.

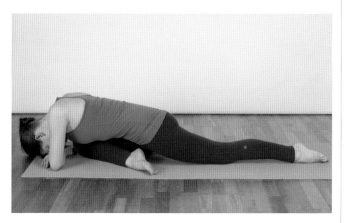

4 Hold for 3–5 deep breaths and change sides.

Hamstring Stretch

Aim: To stretch the back of your leg and release lower back strain.

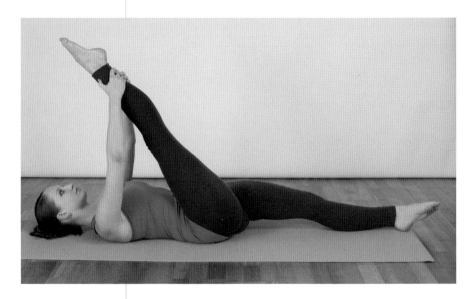

1 Lie flat on the floor, arms by your sides.

2 Lift your right leg and grab hold of your ankle or calf. Keeping your leg straight, use your arms to draw it closer to your body. Keep your tailbone anchored to the floor to activate the stretch fully.

Progression:

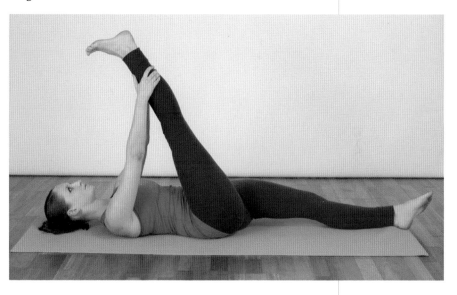

To deepen the stretch, flex your right foot.

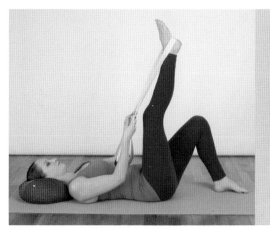

Modification:
If your hamstrings are tight, or you want a lighter stretch, bend your knee slightly. You can also use a strap as pictured. Loop the strap around your foot and pull the ends to draw the leg toward you. A cushion under your head will provide additional support for your neck.

Hamstring Tension Fascia Latae (TFL) Stretch

Aim: To stretch the outer leg and hip, and release lower back and lateral knee tightness.

Helpful Hints:
Keep your pelvis sunk heavily into the floor so that it anchors the hip you are stretching.

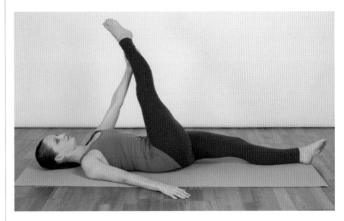

1 From the Hamstring Stretch (see page 152), take the outside of your right foot with your left hand and draw your leg diagonally across your torso toward your left shoulder. Take 5 deep breaths, deepening the stretch with each exhalation.

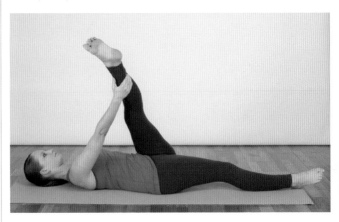

2 Repeat on the opposite side.

Modifications:
For a variation, or if your hamstrings are tight, try a Piriformis stretch instead: keep your knee bent and your foot relaxed throughout the movement. Aim to draw your knee towards the opposite shoulder. You will feel this stretch in your hip and outer thigh.

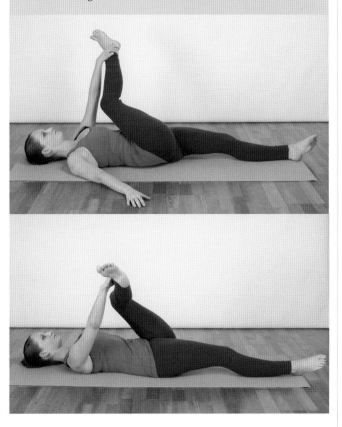

Full Spine Twist

Aim: To release tension in your spine.

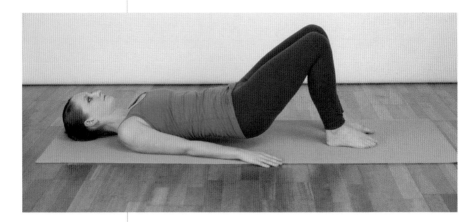

1 Lie on your back with knees bent and feet on the floor. Lift your hips up and shift them over to the left.

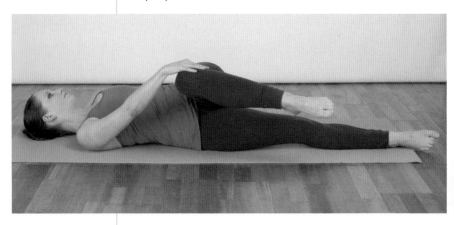

2 Straighten your right leg and roll your left knee over to the right.

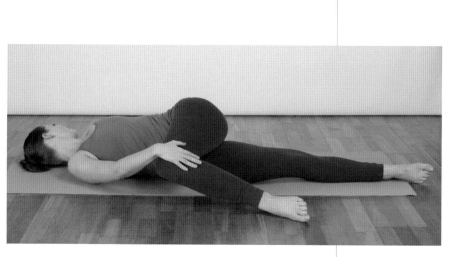

3 Hold the outside of your left knee with your right hand and reach your left hand out to the left.

4 Stay here for 5 deep breaths and then gently come back to center.

5 Return your hips to the middle and stay here for a breath before shifting your hips to the right in order to stretch to the left. Again, stay for 5 breaths and gently return to center.

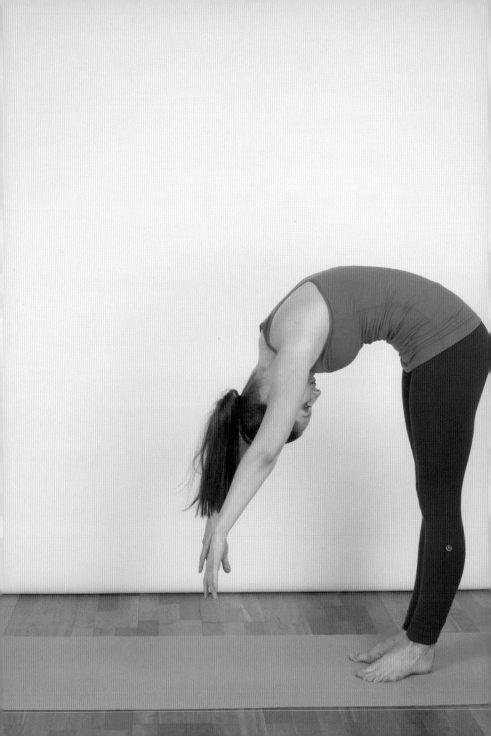

Full Mat Routine

As you approach this section remember that Pilates is a system. As such, it works when the whole of your body is addressed by the entire system of Pilates. Doing this routine in full will give you a full body workout, as well as a block of time to let yourself relax and to be mindful of your body. This is an intermediate level routine, so if you come across a sequence that's outside your comfort zone, try to make the movements smaller.

Breathing Preparation

Aim: To settle your nervous system and draw a line between the rest of your day and your "me time" with your exercise routine.

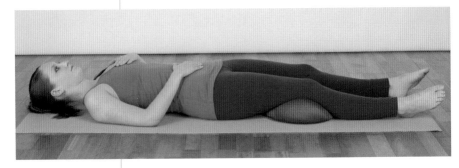

1 Lie down on your back and press the weight of your body fully into the mat.

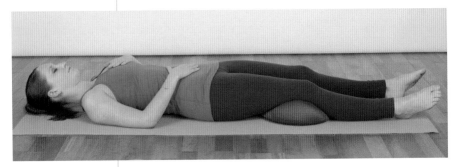

2 Take as many soft, full breaths as you need to feel that you've rid your body of any extraneous tension and mental chatter.

Helpful Hints:
You many find it helpful to breathe in long and gently through your nose, and breathe out through your mouth with a sigh.

Cat Stretch

Aim: To release spine extensors and counterbalance exercises such as the Swan Dive (see page 192).

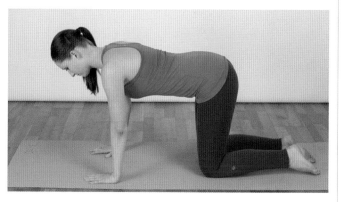

1 Kneel on all fours with your shoulders over your hands and hips over your knees, feet relaxed.

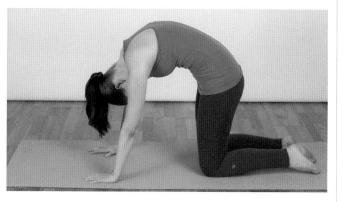

2 Exhale and press into the floor with your hands and knees in order to arch your spine. Inhale to release your spine back to a relaxed position.

3 Repeat 3 times.

161

Knee Hugs

Aim: To begin to co-ordinate breath and movement, and release your lower back.

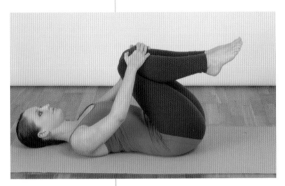

1 Lie on your back with your knees drawn up toward your chest. Feel the weight of your tailbone resting on the floor (if you can).

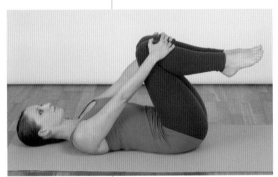

2 As you inhale deep into your belly, float your knees away from your chest until your arms are straight. Imagine the air reaching all the way down to your tailbone and lower belly as you breathe in.

3 Exhale and draw your knees closer to your chest—think of your knees gently squeezing the breath out of your body. Don't let your shoulders tense to squeeze your knees in. Use the strength of your arms and be patient. You will increase your flexibility more by working with your breathing than by forcing things.

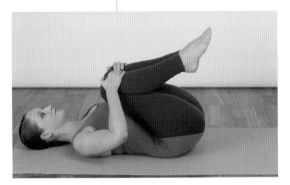

4 Repeat 3 times.

Hip Rolls

Aim: To increase the mobility through your spine and hips.

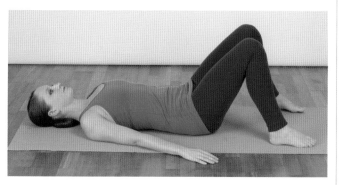

1 Lie on your back with your knees bent, feet flat on the floor wider than your hips, and arms comfortably out to the sides.

Helpful Hints:
• Keep your legs as heavy and passive as possible.
• You should feel a stretch from your top knee through to your hip and lower back. This stretch may extend up to shoulder height.

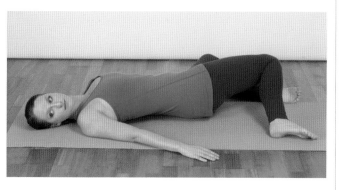

2 Allow your knees to fall gently to the left. Roll your head to the right at the same time. Return to center.

3 Allow your knees to fall to the right. Roll your head to the left at the same time. Return to center.

4 Repeat 3 times to each side.

163

Hundreds

Aim: To stabilize your torso, increase blood flow and challenge your breathing in preparation for larger and stronger movements.

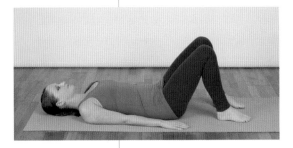

1 Lie on your back with your knees bent and feet flat on the floor. Extend your arms down by your sides and relax your body weight into the floor.

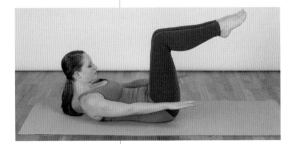

2 Lift your legs into tabletop position.

3 Lengthen your head and upper body into a C-curve, reaching your hands past your hips. Start pumping your arms, breathing in for 5 pumps and out for 5 pumps.

4 Stay in this shape and keep pumping until you have reached 100 pumps (10 times breathing in and out).

Modifications:

• Roll your head and shoulders down, or put your feet back on the floor, but keep pumping and breathing. Gradually, you'll build enough endurance to stay for the whole set.

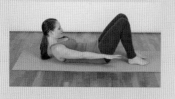

• If you have existing neck problems, learn this exercise with your head down or on a cushion and concentrate on your breath and the pump of your arms to get your blood flowing.

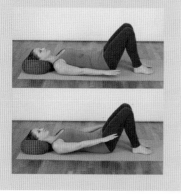

Progression:

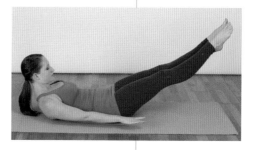

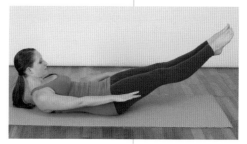

Extend your legs to 45 degrees or even lower with control from your abdominal muscles.

Roll Up

Aim: To articulate your spine and challenge your pelvic and shoulder stability.

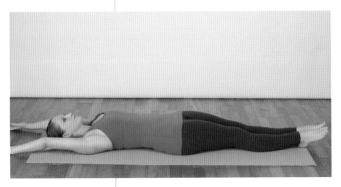

1 Lie on your back with your legs extended out on the mat and your arms stretched out above your head.

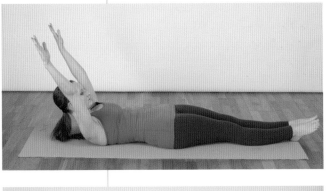

2 Inhale and begin lifting your arms first, followed by your head, neck, and shoulders until you are in a C-curl.

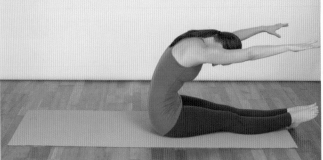

3 Exhale to continue the movement, rolling all the way with your hands reaching for your toes.

Helpful Hints:
Lengthen the front, sides, and back of your spine as you roll.

4 Inhale to begin rolling back down from your sacrum, or tailbone. Articulate all areas of your spine including your neck and lower back.

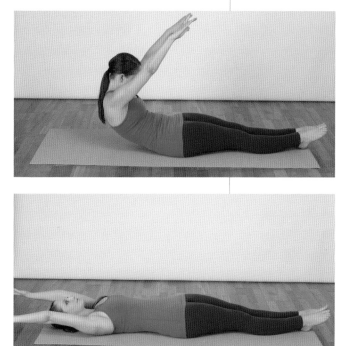

5 Exhale to continue articulating your spine down into the mat, and reach your arms over your head just off the mat.

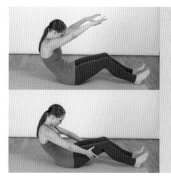

Modification:
• Bend your knees, flex your feet, and keep your heels pressing into the mat as you roll.
• Use your hands on the backs of your thighs to assist in rolling up and down.

167

Roll Over

Aim: To strengthen abdominal muscles and create control via upper body stability.

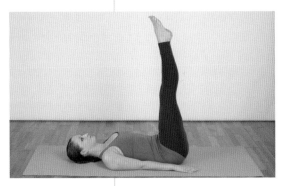

1 Lie on your back with your legs together, stretched up toward the ceiling.

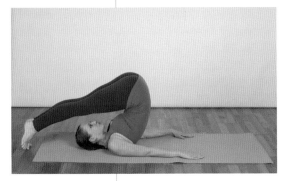

2 Take a breath in and as you breathe out, press your hands into the floor either side of your hips and roll your legs over your head.

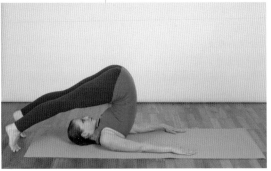

3 Inhale and separate your feet to shoulder width.

4 Exhale to roll back down through your spine.

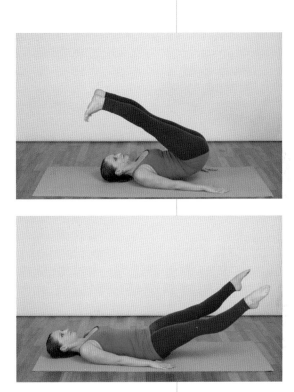

5 Repeat this 3 times and then reverse the "circle" of your legs so that you roll up with your feet shoulder width apart, and roll down with them together.

One Leg Circle

Aim: To articulate your thigh bone in the hip socket and stabilize the pelvis.

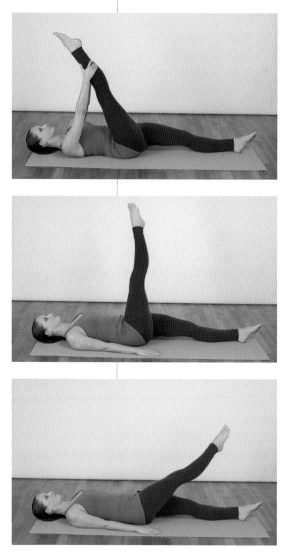

1 Lie down on your back, extend your right leg toward the ceiling, grasp behind your (ideally straight) leg and draw it into your chest for a count of 5.

2 When you release your leg, aim to keep it straight but if your hamstrings don't allow that, bend your knee but keep your thigh vertical.

3 Take 5 circles with your right leg, first crossing the midline, lowering your leg, opening it out to the right and returning to start.

4 Reverse the direction of the circle for 5 repetitions.

5 Change to the other leg and repeat the sequence from the hamstring stretch.

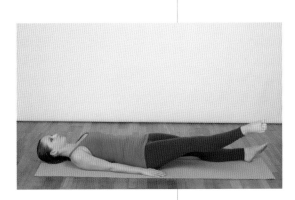

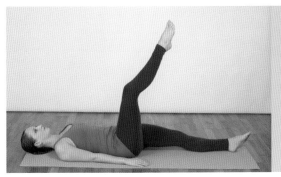

Modification:
Keep your knee bent and make a square instead of a circle to familiarize yourself with the movement.

Progression:
Make the circle bigger. The hip of your circling leg may come off the floor when you cross the midline but make sure your stabilizing hip stays down.

171

Rolling Like a Ball

Aim: To massage and relax the spine, increase breath capacity, develop symmetry and abdominal control.

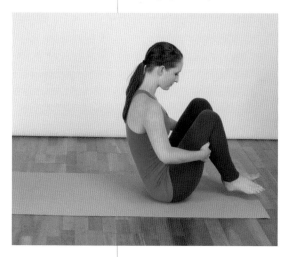

1 Sitting at the front of your mat, draw your knees in and take hold of the back of each thigh. Keep the inside edge of your feet touching and separate your knees to shoulder width.

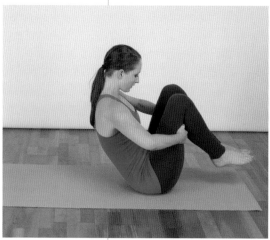

2 Curl your spine back so that you have as much space at the front of your hips as possible and you're drawing your nose toward your knees. You will be sitting, balanced, on the back of your pelvis. Draw your shoulders down to elongate your neck.

172

3 Inhale to roll back until your shoulder blades are just touching the mat and your hips are suspended.

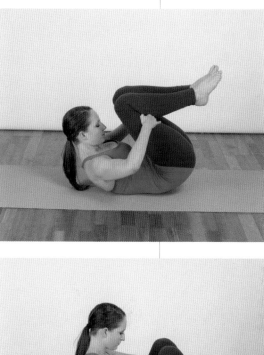

4 Exhale to come straight back up to your balance point.

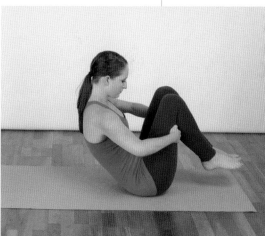

Helpful Hints:
• Keep the tension between your hands and thighs—press one against the other to maintain the "ball" shape throughout.
• Keep your heels close to your bottom to avoid using momentum.

173

Single Leg Stretch

Aim: To challenge center line balance and co-ordination, and increase abdominal control, endurance, and pelvic stability.

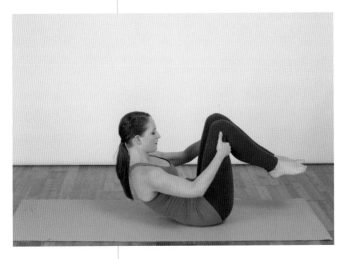

1 Lie on your back with your upper body lifted in a C-curve and your legs in tabletop position.

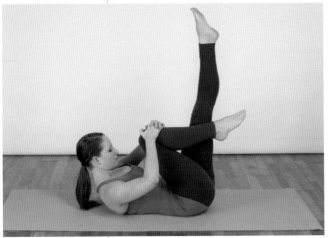

2 Place both hands on your right knee and extend your left leg up toward the ceiling. Your pelvis must stay relaxed in neutral.

174

3 Exhale to switch legs, drawing the bent leg deep into your chest for a back release.

4 Keep switching legs, exhaling as you hug your knee into your chest. Repeat 10 times alternating legs.

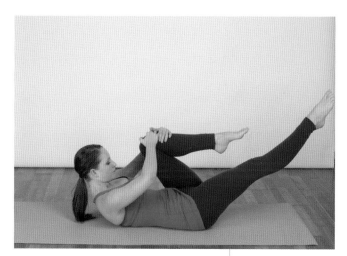

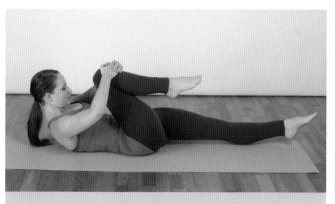

Progression:
Drop your extended leg a little farther away from you for more challenge—keep your pelvis and lower back stable at whatever height you choose.

175

Double Leg Stretch

Aim: To further challenge abdominal muscles, stabilization of pelvis and shoulder girdles and co-ordination between upper and lower body.

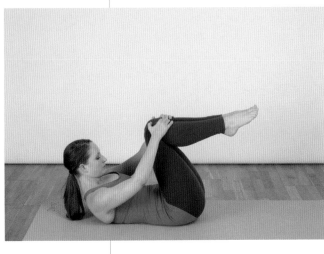

1 Lie on your back with your upper body lifted into a C-curve and your legs in tabletop position.

2 Hold your shins and draw both knees a little more toward your chest.

3 Stay in the C-curve keeping your sacrum anchored into the mat. Inhale and reach both arms and legs up to the ceiling.

4 Exhale and return to the C-curve as you grab your shins. Repeat 10 times.

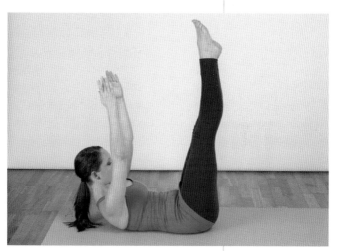

Progression:

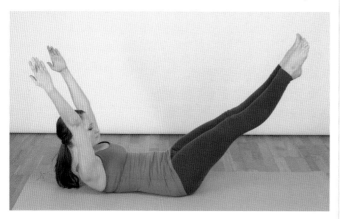

Helpful Hints:
Take your arms and legs an equal distance away from the midline.

Increase the distance of your arms and legs from the midline without sacrificing your C-curve.

177

Scissors

Aim: To challenge abdominal muscles, with stabilization of pelvis and co-ordination between upper and lower body, left and right hand sides.

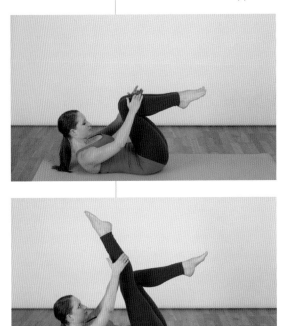

1 Lie on your back with your upper body lifted into a C-curve and your legs in tabletop position with one hand resting on each knee.

2 Extend your right leg toward the ceiling and take both hands around your calf, or if you can't reach it, your thigh. Use the tightness of your hamstrings to keep you in a high C-curve.

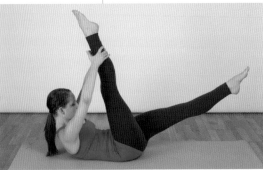

3 Exhale and draw your right leg in toward you, pulse it toward you again.

4 Inhale lightly as you change legs. Exhale to grab and pulse your left leg in toward you.

5 Alternate 10 times.

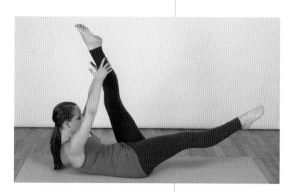

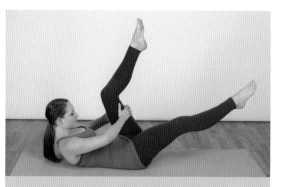

Modifications:
• Keep your legs bent and hold your thigh instead of your calf if your hamstrings do not allow for the full range of movement.
• Alternatively, keep your head down or on a pillow to release your neck.

179

Lower and Lift

Aim: To maximally challenge your ability to maintain pelvic stability against lifting and lowering legs.

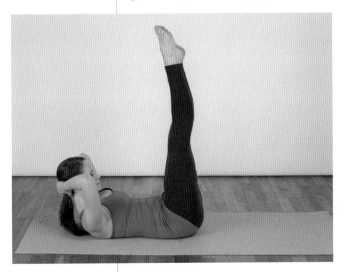

1 Lie on your back with your legs together, stretched up toward the ceiling. Interlace your hands behind your head and curl up into a C-curl.

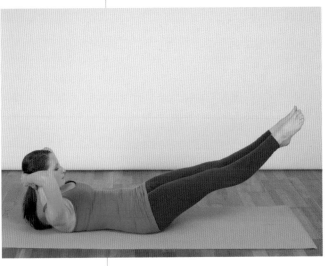

2 Inhale and lower your legs only as far down as you can without your spine starting to arch. If it's simply too hard, try bending your knees to make the lever shorter.

3 Exhale and bring your legs back up to the starting position.

Progression:
You're aiming to go all the way down to the mat—that's challenge enough for anyone!

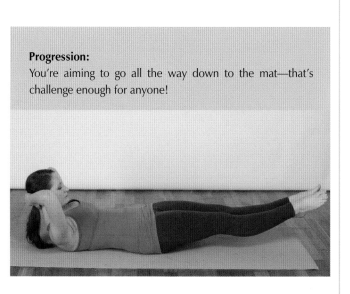

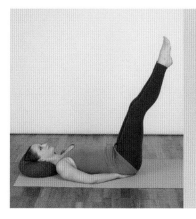

Modifications:
• If you need to release your neck, bring your head down or rest on a pillow and keep your hands behind your head.
• Or try placing your hands under your sacrum. Your hands will provide a fulcrum which makes the exercise easier, but you still have to watch your range to prevent your lower back extending. You can do this alternative either in a C-curl or flat.

181

Criss Cross

Aim: To challenge endurance of whole abdominal group with co-ordination and control of entire body.

Helpful Hints:

• Aim to leave your knee where it is so that you really have to reach with your upper body to get there.

• Aim your bottom elbow to reach behind you rather than being a pivot point on the floor.

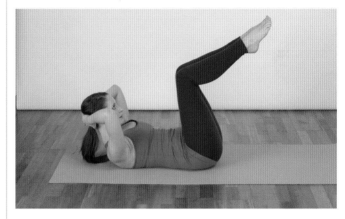

1 Lie on your back with your legs in tabletop, your hands interlaced behind your head, and your upper body lifted into a C-curl.

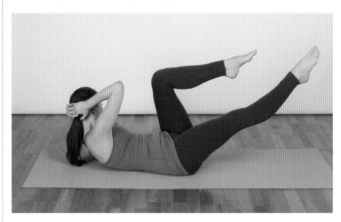

2 Exhale as you rotate to the left aiming your right armpit toward your left knee whilst simultaneously reaching your right leg out to 45 degrees. Inhale to come back to center.

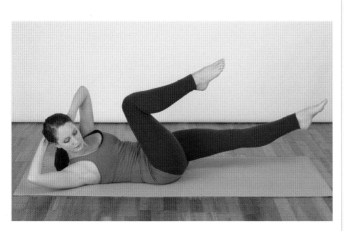

3 Exhale to rotate to the other side, switching legs as you go.

Modification:
Work in a smaller range or keep your knees bent with your feet flat on the ground.

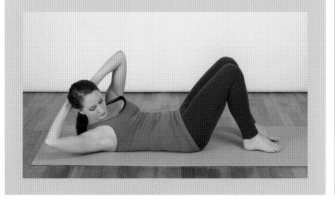

183

Spine Stretch Forward

Aim: To articulate your spine in a seated position. To learn to create space between your vertebrae in movement.

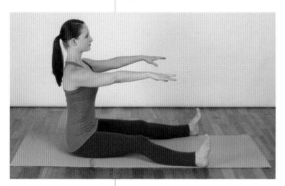

1 Sit tall with your legs outstretched in front of you and your feet hip-width apart. Reach your hands out in front of you at shoulder height, or just below if that creates shoulder tension.

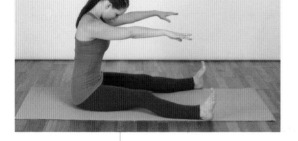

2 Inhale to grow as tall as you can through your spine and begin to nod your head.

Helpful Hints:
Keep sitting firmly on your pelvis throughout rather than letting your hips tip forward. This will require more abdominal lift and encourage more length in your lower back.

3 Exhale to continue to roll down through your spine, thinking of lengthening and articulating the sections of your spine as you move.

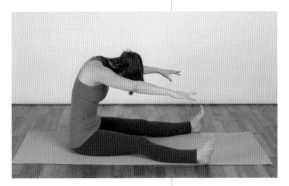

4 Inhale to roll back up through your lower back, middle back, upper back, and neck until sitting tall.

5 Repeat 5 times.

Modifications:
• If the start position is not possible, bend your knees or sit on a cushion to lift your hips up.
• If you're really tight and still can't get your spine upright, sit on a chair as in the desk version.

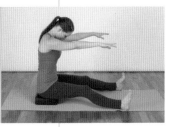

185

Open Leg Rocker Preparation

Aim: To Increase balance, stability and co-ordination in a seated position.

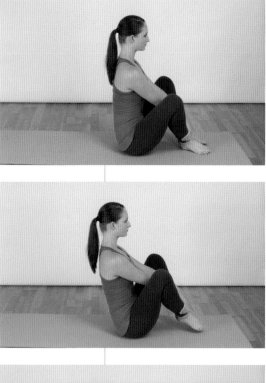

1 Sit with your knees bent and feet flat on the floor. Reach your hands between your legs and grasp the tops of your ankles.

2 Rock onto the back of your pelvis to bring your feet off the floor, keeping them together and your knees shoulder-width apart.

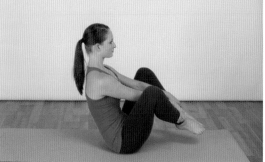

3 Curl your lower body into a C-curl and keep your chest lifted and open.

4 Inhale and straighten one leg as much as possible without moving anything else. Exhale and return to the starting position, feet touching.

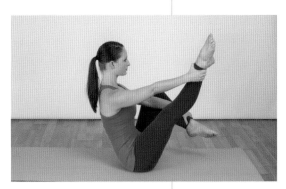

5 Inhale to straighten the other leg and exhale to return.

6 Repeat 3 times on each side.

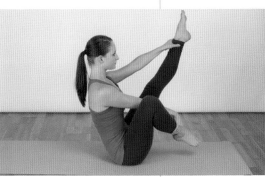

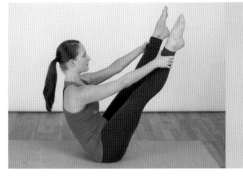

Progression:
For the Open Leg Rocker take both legs out simultaneously, hold for a count of 10 and return simultaneously.

187

Corkscrew

Aim: To strengthen abdominal muscles and create control through upper body stability.

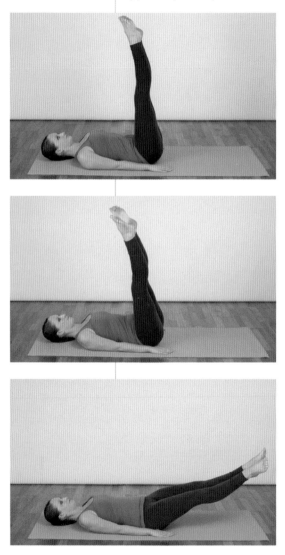

1 Lie on your back with your arms long by your sides and legs together, extended up to the ceiling.

2 Inhale as you circle your legs across to one side.

3 Circle your legs down and away from you.

4 Exhale and bring them across to the other side and back in toward you.

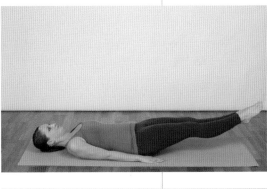

5 Reverse the direction of the circle.

6 Repeat circling one way and then the other for 6 corkscrews.

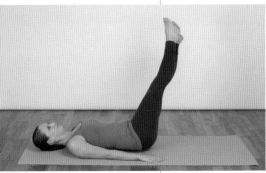

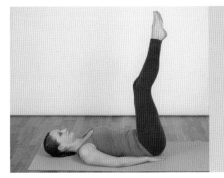

Modification:
• Bend your knees to keep your tail bone on the mat.
• If you need more help, place your hands under your sacrum to provide a platform for the corkscrew.

189

Saw

Aim: To simultaneously stretch and strengthen the torso. Encourage space between vertebrae and strengthen respiratory system.

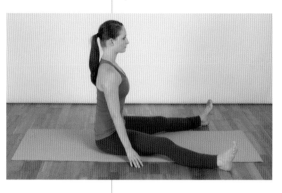

1 Sit with your spine elongated and legs extended out in front of you with your feet as wide as the mat.

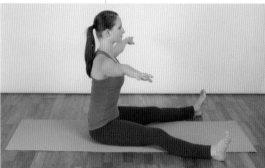

2 Spread your arms to the sides at shoulder height reaching out for as long a span as possible without strain.

Modification:
Sit on a block or on a chair with bent knees, if your hamstrings are limiting your ability to articulate your spine.

3 Inhale to rotate around to the right letting your eyes glide across the horizon until you are facing your right leg.

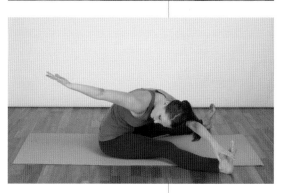

4 Articulate your spine into a curl over your leg as you reach the outside of your left hand to your right little toe. Allow the twist forward bend and percussive breaths to squeeze the air out of your lungs so that as you sit up you naturally take in a full fresh new breath.

5 Exhale with three short percussive breaths as you "saw off" your little toe. Slowly inhale deeply as you return to start position.

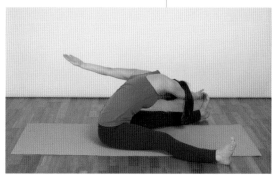

6 Repeat to other side and alternate for 6 in total.

Swan Dive Preparation

Aim: To lengthen and strengthen your spine in extension. Counterbalance the Swan Dive by performing Cat Stretch (page 161).

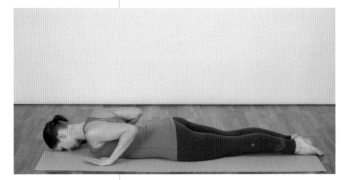

1 Lie on your front with your legs extended, palms down at chest height and elbows pointing up and back.

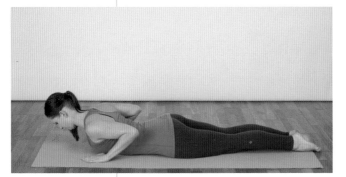

2 Inhale and press down into your hands to extend your spine.

3 Roll up by lifting your chest and articulating your middle back. Lengthen your lower back until your pubic bone begins to lift off the floor.

4 Keep your neck soft by thinking of reaching through the top of your head rather than your nose.

5 Exhale to roll back down. Repeat 3 times.

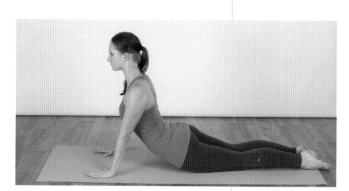

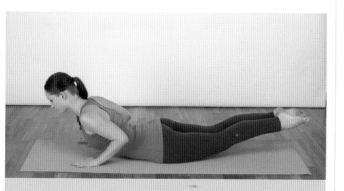

Progression:
• Prepare for the full Swan Dive by adding a double leg lift when you roll down. Lower back must be supported by strong legs, glutes, and abs.
• Think of lengthening both legs away from you as much as possible, keep your pubic bone down and lift your legs. Hold for a count of 3 and lower your legs ready to lift again.

Shoulder Bridge

Aim: To strengthen gluteus muscles, stabilize your pelvis, and challenge torso alignment.

Helpful Hints:
• Keep your weight on your shoulders and not your neck.
• Keep squeezing your inner thighs toward the midline and your hips on the same transverse plane throughout.

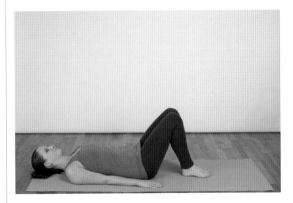

1 Lie on your back with your legs together, knees bent, feet flat on the floor, and arms long by your sides.

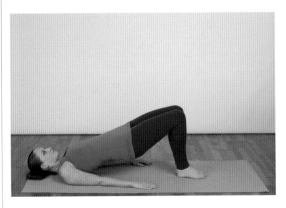

2 Inhale and press your hips up until your head, pelvis, and knees describe a diagonal line.

194

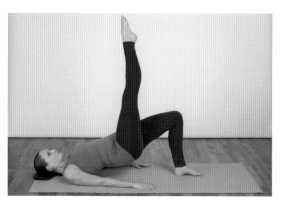

3 Exhale and unfold your right leg to reach to the ceiling.

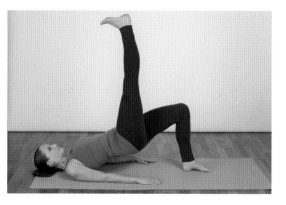

4 Keep breathing naturally while you point and flex your foot 3 times. Inhale and fold your leg back down.

5 Repeat sequence to the other side. Exhale, roll down to the mat, and repeat 3 times.

Side Kick Series

Aim: To tone and strengthen the gluteus muscles and outer thigh, mobilize the hip joint, and challenge torso stability.

Setup:

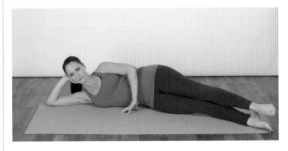

Lie on your side with your head, shoulders, and pelvis in a straight line, and both legs outstretched and angled 45 degrees in front of your trunk. Turn your legs out so that your heels are touching, and your knees are turned away from each other. "Stack" your hips so that your top hip is directly above your bottom hip. Prop your upper body up on your elbow and rest your head in your hand. Rest your other hand in front of your chest—for balance, not strength.

Up Down Top Leg

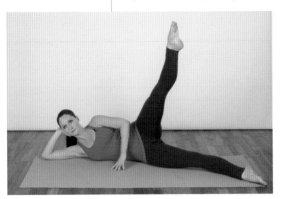

Aim: To tone and strengthen the gluteus muscles and outer thigh, mobilize the hip joint, and challenge torso stability.

1 Assume the set up position shown above.

2 Exhale to kick your leg straight in line with your ear.

3 Inhale, lower your legs, and repeat 10 times.

Progression:
Put your top hand behind your head for more challenge to your stability.

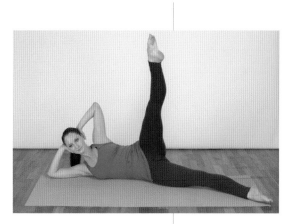

Front Back Top Leg

Aim: To tone and strengthen the glutes and outer thigh, mobilize the hip joint, and challenge torso stability.

1 Assume the set up position shown opposite.

2 Exhale and hinge at your hip to kick your top leg forward, but only as far as you can go with your pelvis remaining in the starting position.

3 Inhale to lengthen your leg into hip extension.

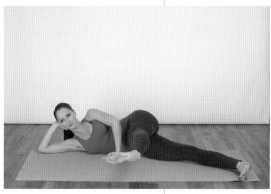

Modification:
• Work in a smaller range to keep hips stable.
• Lie your upper body down and rest your head on your outstretched arm.

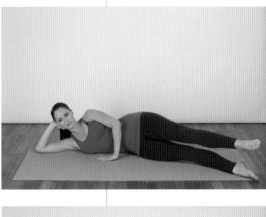

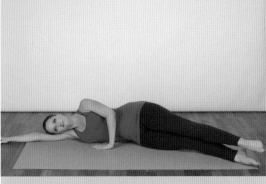

Modification:
• Work in a smaller range to keep hips stable.
• Lie your upper body down and rest your head on your outstretched arm.

Circles Top Leg

Aim: To increase endurance and tone of the hip and gluteus muscles and challenge torso stability.

1 Assume the set up position shown on page 196.

2 Lift your top foot a fraction and circle your leg so that you draw a small controlled circle that goes as far forward as it does backward. Touch your top heel to your bottom heel during each circle.

3 Perform 5 circles each way.

198

Up Down Bottom Leg and Circles Bottom Leg

Aim: To tone and strengthen the inner thigh and challenge torso stability.

1 Assume the set up position shown on page 196.

2 Take your top ankle with your free hand and put your foot in front of your bottom thigh. Ensure your hips are "stacked" so that your top hip is directly above your bottom hip.

3 Exhale and lift the bottom leg reaching it out as far away from your head as possible.

4 Inhale and lower the leg until it just touches the ground and then pick it straight up again.

5 With your leg still lifted, describe a small controlled circle that goes as far forward as it does backward and as far up as it does down.

6 Circle 5 times each way.

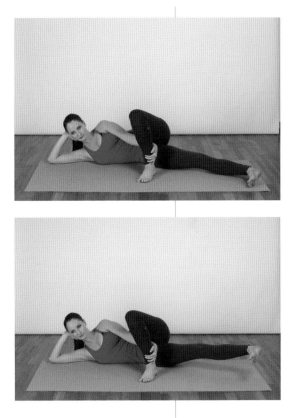

Helpful Hints:
Flex your bottom foot and stretch it away from you both as you lift and as you circle.

Beats

Aim: To release tension in the hips and strengthen abdominal muscles to support the lower back when extended.

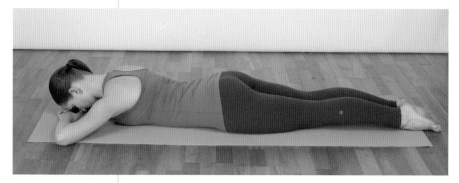

1 Lie on your front with your hands making a rest for your forehead. Reach your legs out behind you, turn your legs out and lightly squeeze your heels together.

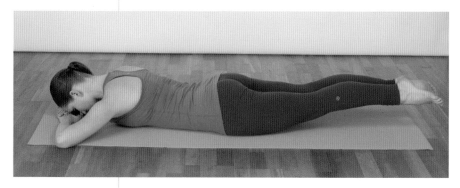

2 Press your pubic bone into the floor and float your legs off the floor.

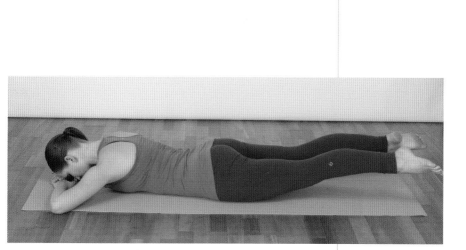

3 Open your feet to hip width and close your legs again, beating your heels together. Breathe in for 5 beats. Breath out for 5 beats.

4 Keep beating and breathing just as for the Hundreds exercise (see page 164) until you have completed 10 breaths (10 times breathing in and out to make a total of 100 beats).

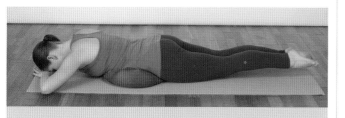

Modification:
Put a pillow under your hips to reduce the load on your lower back.

Teaser

Aim: To increase the difficulty of abdominal control, spinal articulation, and challenge to maintain the length of the spine.

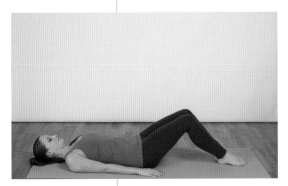

1 Lie on your back with your legs together, knees bent, and feet flat on the floor.

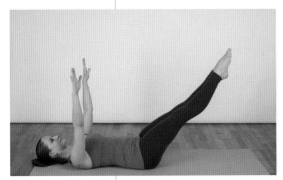

2 Extend your legs to 45 degrees and reach your arms up to the ceiling. Keep your shoulders back as you reach up to the ceiling.

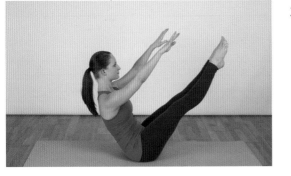

3 Inhale and roll up past your knees, reaching for your toes.

4 Then reach to the ceiling in a smooth movement. Pull into your center line as you move throughout the exercise.

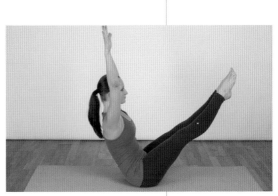

5 Roll back down, articulating through your spine, and with your arms still reaching up so they finish up just off the floor above your head.

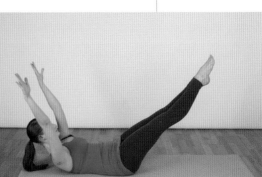

Modifications:
• Keep your arms reaching forward rather than up to the ceiling.
• Bend your knees and keep your legs in tabletop position.
• Use your hands to assist by walking up your legs.
• Extend only one leg to 45 degrees and complete the exercise with 3 repeats to each leg. Repeat 3 times each side.

Swimming

Aim: Simultaneous challenge of pelvis and shoulder stability. Increase endurance for spinal extensors.

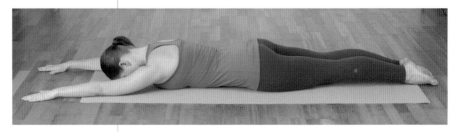

1 Lie on your front with your arms and legs outstretched at shoulder and hip width respectively. Look straight down to the floor so that your neck is long.

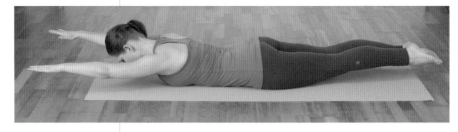

2 Inhale and float your arms and legs off the floor, thinking of reaching up through your head, tail bone, hands and feet rather than lifting up.

Helpful Hints:
• Keep the feeling of your arms and legs staying anchored in your torso even as they reach away.
• Keep your breathing fluid throughout and maintain midline integrity.

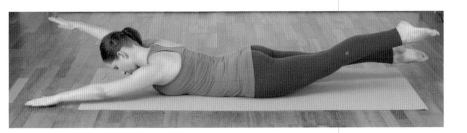

3 Exhale as you alternately lift and lower opposite arm and legs, switching 5 times.

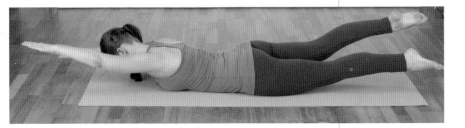

4 Inhale and continue "swimming" with alternate arm and leg kicks for 5 beats.

5 Continue as for Hundreds (see page 164) until you have completed 10 breaths (100 kicks).

Leg Pull Front

Aim: To strengthen shoulders, torso alignment, and whole body co-ordination.

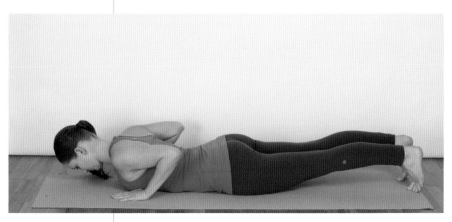

1 Lie on your front with your hands under your shoulders, legs together and outstretched, with your feet flexed so you are propped up with your toes pointing forward. Keep your head in line with your spine and your midline strong.

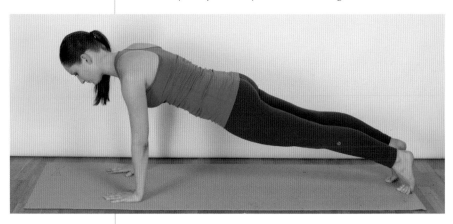

2 Inhale and push your body up into a plank position.

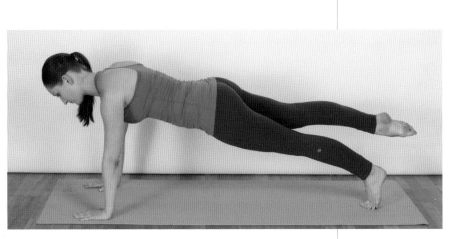

3 Lift one foot off the mat, pointing your toes. Then deeply flex the supporting foot and come back to this position. This should rock your plank forwards, then back. Put your foot down and change legs. Once your second leg is lifed and toes pointed, flex and point the supporting foot then put your foot down again.

Alternate legs 6 times and breathe fluidly throughout

Modification:
• If the plank position is challenging enough without lifting a leg, stay here for a count of 10, then lower to the mat.
• If you are not feeling strong in your upper body, start this position on your hands and knees and step back into plank. Make sure your shoulders are directly above your hands.

Leg Pull Back

Aim: To strengthen shoulders, torso alignment, and whole body co-ordination.

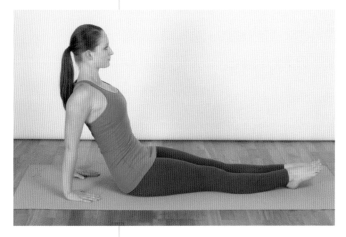

1 Sit on your mat with legs outstretched in front of you and your hands behind you, shoulder-width apart, and with fingers facing forward.

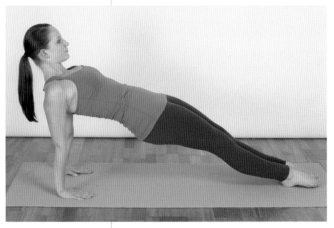

2 Take a breath in and as you breathe out, press your pelvis into the air to create a straight line from your feet through your hips to your head.

3 Exhale and kick one leg to the ceinling without losing control of your hips or shoulders. Inhale to lower down slowly. Repeat 6 times, alternating legs.

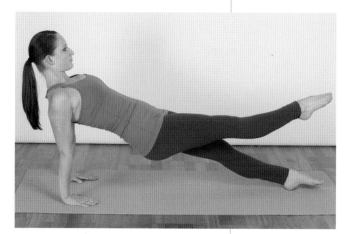

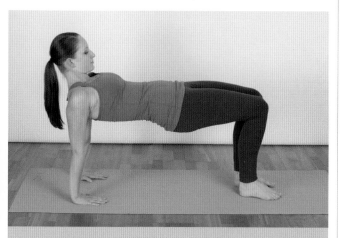

Modification:
Go to Back Support in Revitalize Routine (see page 118).

Side Bend

Aim: To increase shoulder stability, strengthen the respiratory system, stretch and strengthen the sides of the torso.

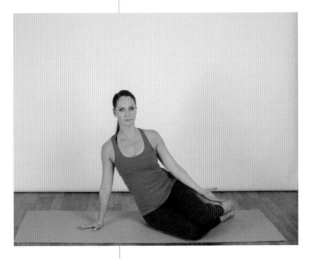

1 Sitting on your right hip, tuck your legs to your left side so that the outside of your right leg is resting on the ground and your left leg is stacked on top. Reach your right hand out in line with your hips and feet and rest your left hand on your left hip with your palm facing up.

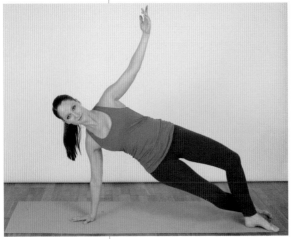

2 Inhale to reach your left hand up toward the ceiling. Simultaneously lift your pelvis and torso into a side bend.

210

3 Continue to push strongly into your bottom (stabilizing) hand to lift and stretch your opposite ribs.

4 Exhale to lower your hips back to the ground and your arm to your side.

5 Repeat 3 times on each side.

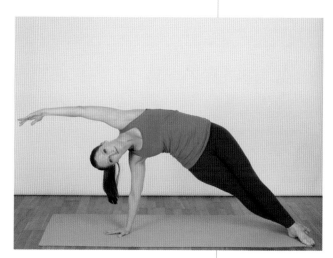

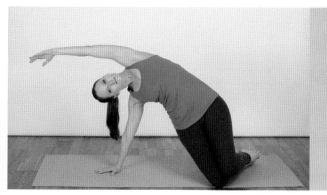

Modification:
Start with your legs in bent position. Use a combination of Mermaid (see page 120) and Side Support (see page 116) to achieve this.

211

Seal

Aim: To release and massage the spine, and challenge balance and co-ordination.

1 Sit with your knees bent and separated to shoulder-width, and your feet touching. Reach through your legs and hold onto the outside of your ankles.

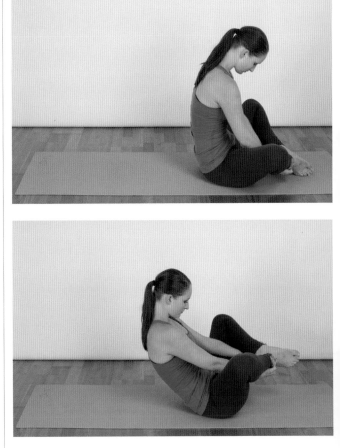

2 Press your thighs into your arms and your arms against your thighs, take your spine into a C-curve, draw your abdominals muscles in, and float your feet off the floor. Clap your feet 3 times, balancing on your sit bones.

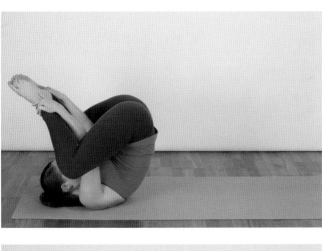

3 Inhale and roll back, reaching your feet over your head towards the mat. Clap your feet and legs together 3 times, balancing on your shoulder blades.

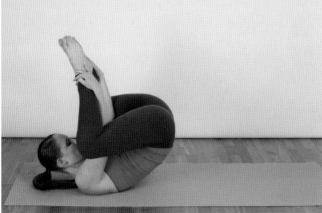

4 Roll back up to clap again.

5 Repeat 5 times.

Push Up

Aim: To challenge whole body organization and upper body strength.

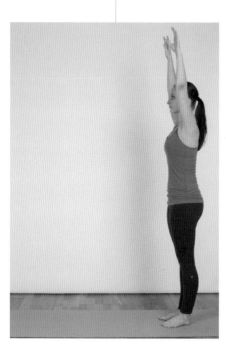 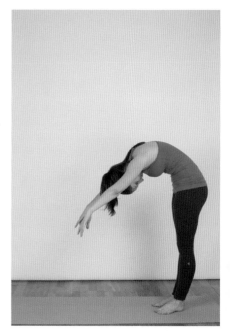

1 Stand with your feet side by side and your arms above your head.

2 Exhale to dive your arms down to the floor.

Modification:
• Bend your knees when you arrive in the plank to perform the push ups.
• Or simply maintain the plank pose for a count of 5–10 before walking back up.

3 Take 3 steps forward with your hands until your body is outstretched with your hands below your shoulders.

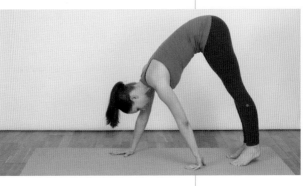

4 Inhale and bend your elbows as much as possible without falling.

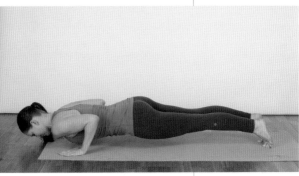

5 Exhale to straighten your arms.

6 Repeat 3 times in total and then walk your hands back in 3 steps.

7 Roll back up to the standing position.

8 Repeat 3 times in total.

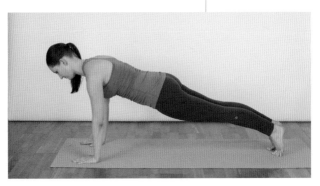

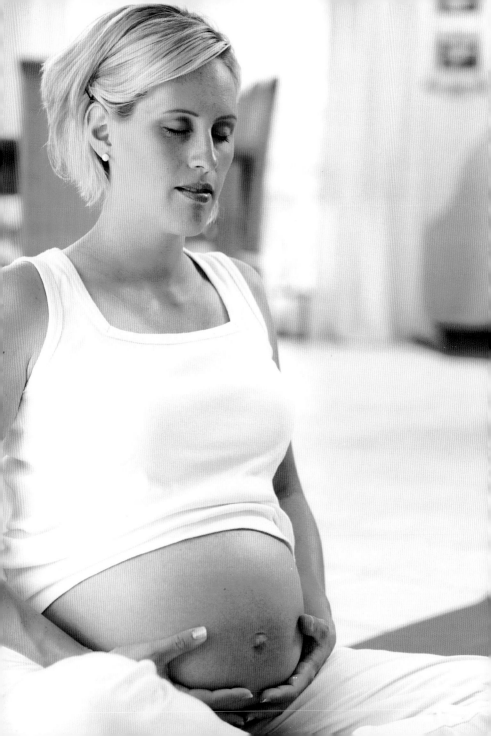

Pilates for Pregnancy

Pregnancy is a state of being, not an illness or an injury, so listen to your body and expect to have to adjust and adapt your routine. The simplest principle to abide by when pregnant is that you can continue whatever fitness or exercise program you were following before you conceived, albeit carefully. Where movements feel comfortable or satisfying, carry on doing them, but when they no longer feel good, stop immediately. In any case, consult your medical practitioner for advice before beginning.

Prenatal Routine

There are many things to take into consideration for the different stages and individual changes during pregnancy when practicing Pilates. Your range of movement in flexing and extending of your spine will be determined by your size, but you can and should move as much as it permits.

Both of the seated At Your Desk routines in this book (see pages 38 and 56) are safe as long as you remain comfortable. See Stressed-Out Shoulders (see page 38) and Lower Back Blues (see page 56). Take care with the Figure 4 Rotation Stretch (see page 62) when you're getting bigger but you probably won't like the feel of it anyway!

Do take particular care when twisting where there is compression in the abdominal area. In all rotations, lift up and visualize the image of the rotation of your upper body (mid-back, shoulders and neck) up and off your baby bump. Lying on your back for any extended period of time is not encouraged in the third trimester. Pay close attention to your body and sit up if you feel any discomfort. If you get dizzy, roll onto your side and take a few moments breathing gently before sitting up.

Use your breath as a reference. Keep your breathing fluid and rhythmic. Avoid holding your breath unless you know exactly what breath practice you are doing and why.

If you have any complications such as SPD (Symphysis Pubis Dysfunction) please seek specialist, personal advice about an exercise routine that is appropriate for you. Consulting your doctor about any exercise routines adopted during pregnancy is always advisable.

Pregnancy Mat Routine

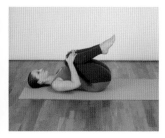

1 Knee Hugs p. 128

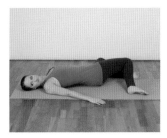

2 Hip Rolls p. 124

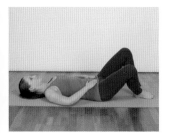

3 The Fan p. 131

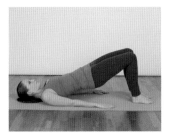

4 Pelvic Press and Roll p. 132

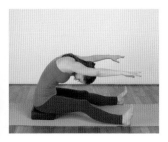

5 Spine Stretch Forward p. 184

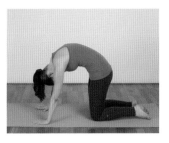

6 Cat p. 161

219

Pilates for Pregnancy

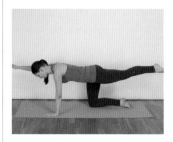

7 Superman p. 144

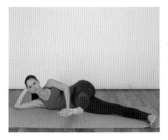

8 Front Back Top Leg p. 197

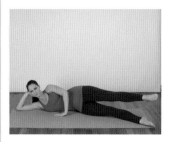

9 Circles Top Leg p. 198

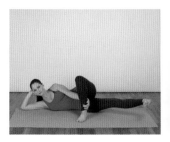

10 Circles Bottom Leg p. 199

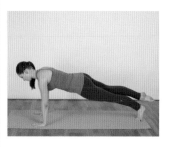

11 Leg Pull Front p. 206

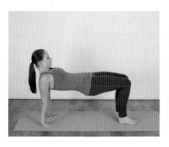

12 Leg Pull Back p. 207

220

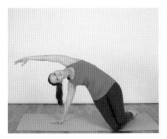

13 Side Bend p. 210

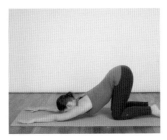

14 Prayer Stretch p. 146

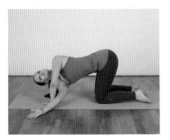

15 Thread Needle p. 148

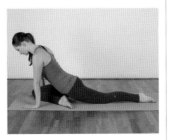

16 Hip Release p. 150

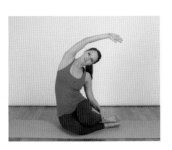

17 Mermaid p. 120

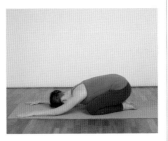

18 Child's Pose p. 147

221

Index

Page numbers in **bold** refer to illustrations.

Index